PALEO DIET FOR BEGINNERS

LOSE WEIGHT AND GET HEALTHY
EATING THE RIGHT FOOD FOR YOUR
BODY +3 WEEKS DIET PLAN

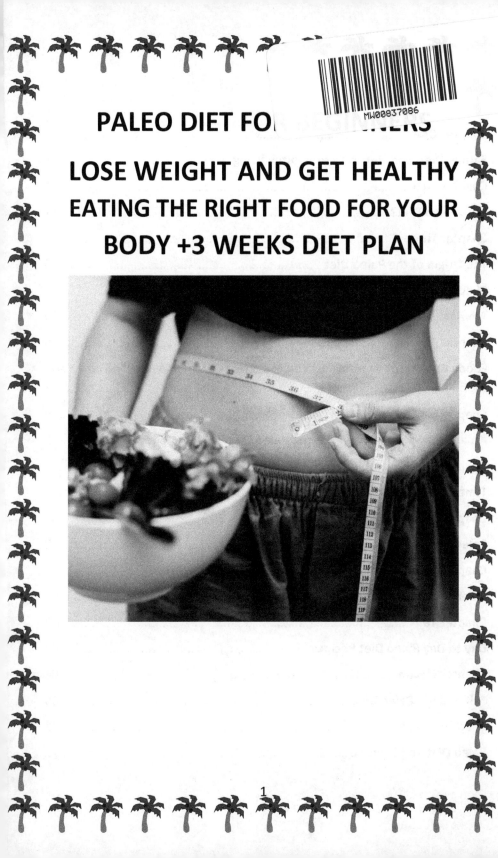

Table of Contents

Introduction

Food is a vital function that provides the essential nutritional elements for good physical, psychological and emotional health. Food is also a social, family and cultural practice that allows you to take a seat in your family and social environment (family meals, outings to restaurants, traditions and religious holidays).

In addition, nutrition plays a preventive role in the onset or development of certain diseases such as obesity, diabetes, high blood pressure or cardiovascular diseases, when it is too rich, too fat or too sweet. It is important to try to maintain a stable weight, which demonstrates a balanced diet. The 3 meals a day (morning, noon and night), allow the person to keep a rhythm of food and a balance of health in the long term, necessary to a healthy and harmonious state of mind.

The diet is individually adapted because the calorie needs vary according to the person, according to their age, their weight, their gender (female or male), their energy expenditure and their physical activity performed. In this book, you will have the opportunity to learn more on how to lose weight and get healthy eating the right food for your body +3 weeks' diet plan. Enjoy the reading!

Chapter One
Eating, Diet, and Nutrition to Healthy living

Nourishing your body is the most natural and essential action of your everyday life. Day after day, every meal involves making food choices, whether conscious or automatic. But do your choices help improve your health and quality of life?

In recent decades, nutrition-related rates of obesity and chronic diseases have increased, although we are becoming more informed about the benefits of good nutrition. There are several factors that can influence your decisions and your eating habits: foods in schools, groceries and restaurants, marketing and social exchanges, or simply lack of information on less nutritious foods.

Collectively, the minds of the population, aging well, is knowing how to keep good health and maintain a physical form in spite of passing years. However, do you think the physical condition is enough to age well? We will see that to experience aging in a positive way it is important to maintain both one's body and one's mind in good health. For that, there are keys like to stay as long as possible active and autonomous and to take general measures concerning their way of life.

The body needs food to function well, for this reason, it is advisable to vary the food in reasonable quantity (eat fruits, vegetables, sugars, fats, legumes, dairy products, meat, eggs, fish, etc.) Water is also very important to the proper functioning of the body. Other drinks, such as coffee, tea, fruit juice, can also be drunk moderately. Also, some foods are known to be beneficial for intelligence, 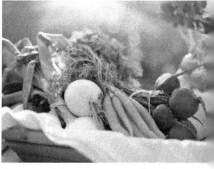 memory, and concentration (fish, all fruits and vegetables, or some food supplements such as wheat, oats, rye, sesame, etc.). On the other hand, it is better to avoid excessive consumption of saturated fats (charcuterie, whole dairy, cheese, butter) and red meats.

At any point in time of one's life, it is essential to engage in daily physical activity as it gives lasting positive health effects, improves quality of life, resistance to fatigue, contributes to the quality of sleep and improves physical fitness.

It should be noted that regular sports practice improves emotional well-being, physical well-being, quality of life (subjective well-being) and self-perception. Studies of the benefits of physical activity show that the risk of premature death is lower in physically active people than in others.

For the adults and the elderly, practicing sporting activities with gentle methods like gymnastics, yoga, walking, is appropriate for keeping muscles and joints in good condition.

However, good food hygiene and the practice of regular physical activity are the first means of prevention to preserve effectively its health capital and to maintain its quality of life and its autonomy.

Being good on your head also helps you feel better. Here are some tips for a healthy lifestyle, which may allow some to reduce the risk of health problems and live more harmoniously:

Have a good philosophy of life:

- Make yourself useful to society and others
- To question oneself to always evolve.
- Enjoy the good moments of life
- Maintain a varied intellectual life by watching the news, reading the newspaper, playing, traveling, staying curious and active
- Ability to stimulate your mind by making memory games, concentration such as Sudoku, Scrabble, arrow words, crosswords, and many others.
- Cultivate your social life: meet new people, go out (go to the cinema, restaurant), be part of an association, etc.

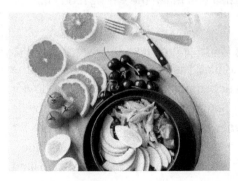

Although our eating habits have a direct impact on our health. A balanced diet is one of the essential components, if not the most essential component, of a healthy life. Many people do not pay much attention to their food choices because they do not realize how powerful food allies can be.

When you eat healthy foods, your body gets the nutrients it needs: vitamins, minerals and fiber, fiber, (healthy) fats, carbohydrates, protein, and these will strengthen the immune system, repair the damage of body, build new healthy cells, recover after an effort and fight against diseases.

The problem with our modern eating habits is that:

1. With our hectic lives, we often end up eating what is practical, rather than what is healthy.
2. Many common foods contain small amounts of nutrients.
3. Fast food, ready meals, and junk food are highly processed. Processing removes a lot of the nutrients, and these foods are often filled with unhealthy ingredients such as chemicals, preservatives, sodium, sugars, and artificial flavors.

Eating these unhealthy foods on a regular basis can cause undernourishment even if you eat a lot of food. And since these are calories without nutritional value, your body does have the nutrients it needs (even if you fill your stomach).

The best choice is to focus on healthy foods. Focus on good foods like fruits and vegetables, beans and legumes, nuts and seeds (whole grains).

The most immediate and visible effect of poor food hygiene on our health is weight gain, and sometimes even obesity. But this is the visible side of the iceberg because then come problems like diabetes, heart disease, high blood pressure, underweight, weak bones, and sometimes even depression or problems cognitive. A multitude of other problems and pathologies not listed here can occur in the medium-long term if you make the wrong food choices. Diet is the key to good health!

Eating well does not just mean eating soups, eating less, or saying no to fat. Healthy eating habits mean a nutritious diet, that is, eating everything in the right amount and in the right way. Do not completely exclude fat and do not overdo it with fiber and protein! Do not forget that you have to provide children with a good balance of all types of foods, because it is the age for physical and mental development. And finally, forget the processed foods, limit to the maximum sugar, salt, white flour, and some might tell you to limit also the cow's milk (the famous 4 whites).

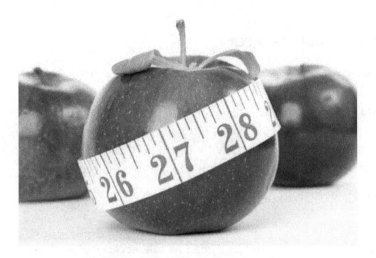

1. MAINTAIN ONE'S FITNESS WEIGHT

Exercising regularly and eating well can help you maintain a healthy weight and avoid getting fat. It is, therefore, preferable to maintain good food hygiene over time rather than trying to catch up with diets. When you stop dieting, you will almost always regain all the weight you have lost. All your efforts to lose weight will have been useless.

2. DISEASE CONTROL

By lowering unhealthy triglycerides and promoting good cholesterol, good dietary choices can prevent many dangerous health problems. Some foods are anti-oxidants and anti-inflammatories, which avoids the damage caused by free radicals. When a diet is healthy, it assists your body to minimize the risk of cardiovascular disease. Obesity, diabetes, cancer, high blood pressure, heart disease, stroke, and osteoporosis are all consequences of poor eating habits.

3. KEEP YOUR BRAIN IN GOOD SHAPE

A diet that is healthy is as good for your brain as it is for the rest of your body system. Unhealthy foods are linked to a whole series of neurological problems. Some nutritional deficiencies increase the risk of depression. Other nutrients, such as potassium, are involved in the functioning of brain cells. A varied and healthy diet keeps your brain functioning and can also promote good mental health.

4. DECREASE THE RISK OF CANCER

Fruits and vegetables are loaded with antioxidants, which are substances that seek out and neutralize potentially harmful cells (free radicals). Free radicals contain an unequal amount of electrons, which makes them very unstable. When they search for and steal electrons in healthy cells, they can cause damage. Antioxidants neutralize the body by freeing radicals and donating one of their electrons, turning the free radical into a stable molecule.

5. CONTROL OF BLOOD GLUCOSE

Sweet foods such as white bread, fruit juice, soft drinks, and ice cream cause a spike in blood sugar. Although your body can handle occasional surges of glucose, over time this can lead to insulin resistance, which can turn into type 2 diabetes. Complex carbohydrates, such as whole grain bread, oatmeal oats, and brown rice, cause a slow release of sugar in the blood, which helps to regulate blood sugar.

6. A LONGER LIFE AND QUALITY

To be healthy, in addition to a healthy diet, you should start exercising, quit smoking, start monitoring your cholesterol levels, your blood pressure, and your weight. Eating healthy is more a part of a lifestyle change than a diet. You will gradually feel the need to feel good about all aspects of your life.

Chapter Two
Why Paleo Diet?

A diet can be followed as a therapeutic or preventive treatment of a disease. Many people decide to diet to refine their silhouette and lose the famous "extra pounds." A diet is prescribed by a doctor to treat health problems therapeutically or preventively. Going on a diet helps to treat, relieve or reduce a patient's symptoms, such as diabetes, cardiovascular risks, overweight, and a food allergy.

Paleo is one of the healthiest ways to eat because it uses a nutritional approach that relies on genetics to keep your body slim, strong and enthusiastic. Research in most food and nutrition expertise and the Paleo review show that this diet is the modern full of refined foods.

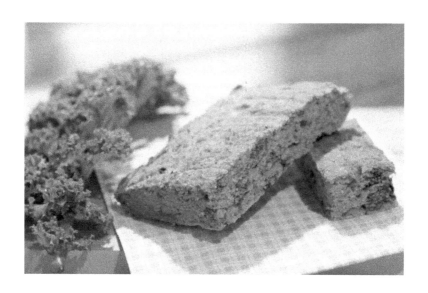

Paleo diet is also called the Caveman diet, Hunter-gatherer diet, Paleolithic diet or Stone Age diet. It's become popular among most lovers of. This usually includes eating what people in the Paleolithic eat, such as lean meats, fruits, vegetables, nuts, and seeds. However, a Paleo diet limits foods such as dairy products, legumes, and cereals.

What Is the Right Choice for You?

Although the Paleo diet is not the best for anyone who does not agree with some of its dietary limitations, it a proven fact that it provides a healthy alternative for those who desire to lose weight and improve their health. General like any other market, this diet must have a balance between all the foods eaten. This program allows you to get all the nutrients the body needs without eating too much. This diet is the perfect choice for you because it is a natural way to lose weight with less risk to your health.

The Paleolithic Diet, also known as the Caveman Diet, is a diet modeled on the eating habits of humans or rather our Homo habilis ancestor of the Paleolithic age that began about 2.5 millions of years. Although the Paleo diet seems new, it was revived several decades ago. It was launched around the 70s by the American gastroenterologist Walter Voegtlin with the idea that our ancestors of the Paleolithic could teach modern men how to eat healthily.

When we eat Paleo, we eliminate all foods containing salt or sugar, or dairy products, cereals, legumes, but also refined oils appeared for 10,000 years. Indeed, our DNA has remained the same since the Paleolithic era, but our diet has changed radically from that time, and things have even accelerated over the past 50 years. The food that we are adapted to, that which allows us to be the fittest and healthy, would be that of the Paleolithic: fresh food from hunting or gathering (meat, fish, poultry, eggs, vegetables and fruits, nuts and seeds, herbs and spices).

Paleo has been known for several years now, but it has never been so seduced. Unlike other diets, it was not "designed" by a nutritionist since it corresponds to what the first humans ate naturally. It is based on the assumption that modern food is not genetically adapted to our species and that we should eat like the first hominids who were "hunter-gatherers." In other words, our genetic heritage has not changed in 40,000 years while food models, they have completely changed, especially since the development of livestock and agriculture in the Neolithic.

It is this shift that gradually introduced degenerative diseases that our ancestors probably did not know. The researchers even think that they would be able to compete with the best modern athletes. Some, like Dr. Jean Seignalet, who died in 2003, have even used this diet against autoimmune diseases such as multiple sclerosis, rheumatoid arthritis or fibromyalgia, three diseases that traditional medicine is struggling to treat.

For several years now, researchers have been striving to identify precisely the composition of this prehistoric regime. Even if no consensus really emerges, researchers agree on different points: during the Paleolithic, dairy products, cereals (including bread) and legumes were not part of it. Salty foods, refined sugar, soft drinks, and processed foods either. On the other hand, it seems that the paleo diet was richer in protein and fat than the modern diet. But unlike the programs richly documented by some books. Beyond the lack of knowledge about the eating habits of our ancestors, the Paleolithic regime, so attractive, comes up against several limits.

As you can see, the paleo diet favors foods available in the Paleolithic era. It, therefore, focuses on quality in the foods you eat because they are fresh, whole, natural and these are the ones that contain more vitamins and minerals. It is the guarantee of better health, mood, recovery, performance and also less risk of injury and inflammation in general.

It is an excellent diet that will bring you many benefits and can be followed by any person (sports or not) wanting to lose fat and regain vitality while being satiated. You understand it; it's not just a "diet" but a way to eat which is synonymous with common sense.

Be aware, however, that we are able to digest certain modern foods (except cases of intolerance) that appeared later on the scale of human evolution. They should not be the basis of your diet but can benefit athletes whose physical activity requires a higher intake of carbohydrates and proteins or simply by the question of taste and desires. These are cereals (preferably gluten-free), legumes (making sure they are soaked), dairy products, preferably raw milk and even some food supplements (protein powder, vitamin D, Omega-3, etc.).

Everything is a question of quantity, if you respect 80% of the main principles of the paleo diet, you will get excellent results. If you do not have enough to eat paleo, do not deprive yourself, do you serve something else that allows you to eat your fill. Do not disorganize, sharing in a group is part of the pleasures of life and therefore well-being. Having a beer or a glass of wine occasionally has never hurt anyone. Conversely, just because you put 2 cherry tomatoes among your fries and there are strawberries in this beautiful " strawberry " ice cream, does not mean that your meal will be balanced. You have understood, everything is a question of balance, be regular, consistent, it is the key.

Nutrition is at the forefront of a healthy body system, and among the most important in your daily life, it is the main lever towards progression and performance, so it must not be neglected or left to chance. It is a vital need that we repeat several times a day and of which your general form will depend completely. So you now know why the paleo regime is at the center of all discussions and in other areas such as health and well-being.

Chapter Three
The Origin of the Paleo Diet

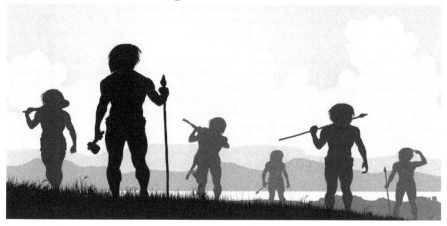

In ancient times, humans survived by hunting, fishing, and harvesting fruit, vegetables, and other products of the earth. This is why many scholars have called these our ancestors "hunter-gatherers". But it is not as immediate as it might seem. The variety of foods depended heavily on areas and seasons. And also by chance, skill and other factors that today would not be important or limiting at all. DNA research has shown that in the last 40,000 years, DNA has changed to a negligible percentage, quantifiable as only 0.02%, making, in fact, the constitution of man practically equal to that of men of the most recent Paleolithic that is Upper Paleolithic.

What Did They Eat?

It is done first to say what they did not eat or, better, what changed between 10,000 and 15,000 years ago (the period changes according to the areas considered). Between 10,000 and 15,000 years ago, a man began to understand that it was possible to avoid migrations linked to the alternation of the seasons and that it was possible to obtain conservable or usable food resources all year round. This possibility was linked to the discovery and adoption of 2 new practices: agriculture and breeding.

Our eating habits and the decrease in physical activity play a decisive role in the emergence, at a pandemic level, of diseases called civilization, for example, coronary heart disease, hypertension, type 2 diabetes, and many others.

Surprisingly, these diseases are absent in the rare contemporary hunter-gatherer populations that have not yet come into contact with the western lifestyle. Their lifestyle seems not to have evolved since the Upper Paleolithic which is around 40,000 years ago.

Some researchers have associated this deplorable current situation with the rapid and frequent changes our environment has undergone for several decades. What is interesting is that unlike our environment and above all the food industry (and therefore of people's food), Our genome (our set of genes) has practically not changed. This leads us to say that socially, we are certainly in the 21st century, but genetically, we have remained in the Upper Paleolithic. Some believe it is this temporal gap between genome and environment that could explain the current rise in civilization diseases. We can partially associate the appearance and growing fame of the Paleolithic diet with these rather rational explanations.

However, not everyone agrees on the facts mentioned above, and numerous variables, as well as the evaluation of the context, must be taken into consideration.

If we take a step back in time, scientific literature reveals that the foods typically consumed during that era were ripe and sweet fruits, berries, meat, fish, crustaceans, insects, larvae, eggs, animal bone marrow, roots, tubers, nuts and seeds other than grasses. Strangely, this type of food provides about 25% of the energy intake of the typical person of our age. This means that now, most of our daily energy comes from seeds, dairy products, sugars, refined fats, and vegetables. On the other hand, the guidelines of some recognized institutions in the field of nutrition and the foundations of

Paleolithic nutrition have several points in common. For example, take less sodium and refined sugars, along with a richer diet of fruit and vegetables.

The techniques used to reconstruct the typical paleo diet of the "ancient humans" are mainly based on the analysis of their teeth, but also the size and confirmation of their jaw. The exploration by anthropologists of the sites where our ancestors used to camp has made it possible to highlight the remains of animal bones and fish they have consumed, as well as the tools used to peel and prepare them. On the other hand, with the new technologies of microscopic dental analysis and chemical analysis techniques, we could have surprises about the variety of our ancestors' nutrition. Furthermore, the relationships between micronutrients (proteins, carbohydrates, and fats) found in their diet seem to vary depending on the historical sites studied and the methods of analysis used.

In addition, the paleo diet or 'evolutionary' diet is an urban legend launched for the first time by the gastroenterologist Walter Voegtlin (The Stone Age Diet, 1975), and taken up in the following years by various authors with studies of a scientific nature. The widely shared narrative indicates that the man would have regulated his genetic heritage, and therefore his physiology, eating mainly lean meat and vegetables during the Paleolithic (period ranging from 2.5 million to 10 thousand years ago). With the advent of agriculture and breeding, and the massive introduction of new foods such as cereals, milk, and derivatives, man would not have succeeded in adapting. Hence the development of diseases typical of civilization, such as obesity, diabetes and tooth decay.

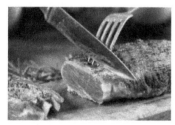

In reality, we do not know how our ancestors ate 1-2 million years ago in the various continents, in different seasons and latitudes. There were probably many 'paleo diets' that varied with the seasons. So we are talking about a food model that existed during our ancestral period.

Since the 1950s, the idea had spread among several anthropologists and even at the popular level, that the evolutionary step of Homo erectus would not be due to the consumption of tubers (some varieties of potatoes), but to the introduction in the diet of the meat (' Man the Hunter hypothesis '). The carcasses of numerous animals found in some caves would confirm this thesis. Unfortunately, the tubers or other vegetable products, being devoid of bones, have left no trace in the evolution of our species.

Several experts since the 1970s have considered this hypothesis a mere conjecture and recent analyses of the dental plaque of remains of Australopithecus sediba (South Africa, 2 million years ago) show that food was very similar to that of many contemporary primates. Nothing to do, therefore, with the supposed diet rich in meat so dear to the followers of the paleo regime.

Furthermore, residues of starch from different types of cereal grains found in archaeological sites 30,000 years ago in some part of the world like Russia, Italy, and the Czech Republic have been found. Therefore, a man introduced cereal starch into his diet long before 10 thousand years ago. Always the analysis of the dental plaque of Neanderthal man (200 thousand-40 thousand years ago) highlights the consumption of foods rich in gelatinized starch, a transformation that takes place only when starchy cereals are cooked.

Without disturbing the paleo nutrition experts, we can safely say that man has never eaten so much meat different from that of the Paleolithic as in recent decades, simply because there were no farms and it was not easy to get hold of it. Moreover, it was easily perishable because the cold chain did not exist, in a word, the refrigerator! Actually, we do not know what has led to the evolution which led to ' H homo sapiens brains of 1,300 cubic centimeters.

The ability to transform food before eating it (a sort of 'pre-digestion'), according to anthropologist Katharine Milton, and the introduction of fire to cook food, according to primatologist Richard Wrangham, have certainly helped to cope with the increased energy demands of the brain. Cooking is able to make perfectly assimilable foods that are not digestible let's think for example of a tuber or a raw potato, practically indigestible. It is not clear at which time the fire was used for cooking food, but some findings suggest 1.7 million years ago.

It is therefore not necessary to look at prehistory (paleo nutrition) to understand what is the ideal diet for humans, since we already know what the best food model is for living long and healthy: a diet based mainly on products of plant origin (plant-based diet) with plenty of cereals or tubers, fruit, vegetables, legumes, nuts, and small amounts of food of animal origin (meat, milk and derivatives, eggs, fish) or Mediterranean diets and vegetarian diets. The scientific evidence is consistent. The science of nutrition also tells us that it is good to avoid highly processed foods from the food industry in order to limit as much as possible the added sugars (sucrose, glucose, fructose, etc.), salt, fats (which increase density food calories) and alcohol (wine, beer, spirits).

Chapter Four
Advantages and Disadvantages of the Paleo Diet

The Paleo diet, also known as the Paleolithic diet or the cave diet, is a diet based on the type of diet that characterized the cavemen who lived some thousands years ago when, before advent of agriculture, human beings fed on the food obtained from practices such as hunting, fishing and harvesting the fruits of the earth that arose spontaneously. According to the proponents of the paleo diet, the human genome has practically not changed since then, while the advent of agriculture has substantially modified the diet of man, causing the health problems that today have exploded: obesity, overweight, diabetes, intolerances, allergies, and many others.

The paleo diet is therefore mainly protein based on the consumption of meat, fish, non-starchy vegetables, fruit, and nuts. The reasons behind the diet lie in the fact that when the Paleolithic age was nourished in this way the risk of running into serious pathologies was quite reduced and in fact the spread of cardiovascular, cancer and metabolic pathologies is strongly related to nutrition modern based on sugars, refined cereals, and junk food.

It should be noted that these foods should be chosen organic and as far as meat is concerned, since the one normally sold is meat stuffed with hormones, it should be consumed grass fed, the meat of cattle fed on grass and not on grains and hormones. The Paleo diet encourages eating less processed foods and more fruits and vegetables. It reduces the consumption of high-calorie foods by reducing the calorie intake and helping you lose weight.

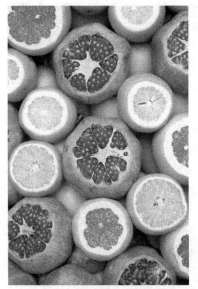

The diet is simple and does not involve counting calories. Some programs start from the "80/20" rule, so, for example, you will get 99% of the benefits if you manage to follow 80% of the time. This flexibility can make the diet easier to deal with, thus making it more likely to succeed.

The fiber intake also helps intestinal transit. The diet provides, for the necessary intake of carbohydrates and sugars, an important consumption of fruit and vegetables, precious sources of vitamins, antioxidants and mineral salts.

The paleo diet can be followed almost everywhere because all foods to eat are readily available. The paleo diet would reduce the level of insulin in the blood, but also cholesterol. The high consumption of fruits and vegetables also has health benefits since it provides multiple vitamins and minerals necessary for the proper functioning of the body.

Among the benefits of the paleo diet, we find the consumption of proteins, which quickly satiate and allow high-intensity physical activities. Another pro is definitely to take a break from all the industrial products we eat when we're in a hurry, or we're bored. No snacks, drinks, ready meals and junk foods. The health of the heart and the liver will certainly benefit.

So What Are the Disadvantage Sides of the Paleo Diet?

Undoubtedly positive is the preference for carbohydrates (albeit with many limitations) with low glycemic content and high fiber content. This allows you to lower the glycemic index and lose weight naturally.

On the other hand, milk and its derivatives are not included in the diet, and therefore, according to Paleo diet detractors, the necessary calcium and vitamin D intake is lacking. Furthermore, it is not always easy, nowadays and considering the development of society and consumption, find meat and fish that are not " treated."

If the Paleolithic diet could have made sense two million years ago it is currently much more difficult to follow it to the letter; it provides for many restrictions, such as the lack of all leavened products, starchy foods, baked goods.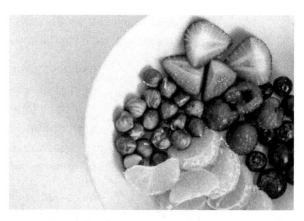

Furthermore, the consumption of mainly raw meat or game does not fall within the tastes of everyone, it is not easy to adapt to the flavor of raw meat or game, not to mention the difficulty nowadays of finding fresh meat suitable to eat raw without the risk to find health damage due to bacterial or parasitic contamination.

We must not forget that primitive man did not at all have a sedentary life: to burn all the fats (30-60%) required by the diet, you need to do some exercise, forget for a while the slippers and the sofa and dedicate at least 30 minutes a day to intense physical activity.

Several nutritionists claim that the Paleo diet is too restrictive and lacking in logic as it excludes whole categories of food by basing consumption on other categories. This way of eating is not balanced and, among other things, there is no scientific basis, according to experts, for which the followers of the Paleo live longer than others or are rarely subject to the onset of some diseases.

The Paleo diet must, however, be adapted to the different needs and if on the one hand, it may seem simple to do alone, on the other it is better to rely on an expert who can follow in the dietary path, especially if there are particular health conditions.

Like any other diet, the Paleolithic diet also shows some disadvantages. There are also some contraindications of the paleo diet. One of the risks is the yo-yo effect: the rapid weight loss in the first weeks and the subsequent vitamin D deficiency.

Like any other weight loss diet, the Paleolithic diet also has a list of permitted and prohibited foods which include:

- Foods permitted in the paleo diet: fruit, vegetables, red meat, white meat, eggs, fish
- Foods prohibited in the paleo diet: legumes, cereals, dairy products, foods with preservatives, sugars
- Foods to be consumed in moderation: oil, tea, café, dried fruit

However, as summer approaches, the desire to feel more beautiful, fit and ready to lose those extra pounds that winter has unfortunately given us is growing. To our rescue, large groups of food experts arrive ready to give us some tips to help us lose weight and finally feel in harmony with the warm season and with ourselves. One of the most popular diets in recent times is the Paleo diet, which refers to the typical diet of the Paleolithic men when neither agriculture nor livestock existed. Disadvantages of the Paleo Diet, meat and fish at will but. In those faraway times, men used to feed themselves with what, thanks to hunting and fishing, Mother Nature put at their disposal: mainly, therefore, meat and fish. Transposed in our times, the paleo diet certainly does not lend itself to being suitable for vegetarians by providing a large consumption of meat and fish in contrast to some of the most current trends that instead advise against the use of them, especially meat.

Another disadvantage of the Paleo diet, nutritional deficiencies banned from the Paleo diet dairy products and whole grains that normally today are part of a healthy and balanced diet. Furthermore, one of the most obvious disadvantages of the paleo diet is that it can prove to be expensive, especially due to the fact that being high in protein, cuts of meat can cost quite a bit. All artificial foods and artificial sweet substances are banned from the paleo diet, with the exception of honey, which must, however, be consumed in moderate quantities. Excluding basic food groups, the risk of nutritional deficiencies increases, which could be expected to compensate by taking food supplements and vitamins.

In addition, there are no accurate records of the diet followed by our Stone Age ancestors, so the Paleo diet is based on hypotheses, and its health claims have no scientific evidence. Most versions of the diet encourage large amounts of meat, which is in contrast to current evidence that discourages consumption.

Many versions prohibit dairy products and whole grains, which instead are part of a healthy and balanced diet. Like all high protein diets, Paleo can be expensive, depending on your choice of meat cuts. It is impossible to do the diet without eating meat, fish or eggs, so it is not for vegetarians.

Most versions of the Paleo Diet exclude basic food groups, increasing the risk of nutritional deficiencies unless careful substitutions are made. Use of food supplements is not excluded. The diet has some positive aspects, so an adapted version that does not prohibit food groups such as whole grains, dairy products and legumes could be a better choice.

This regime requires great rigor because it is very restrictive. Some foods such as bread, pasta, rice, and all other grain products can be difficult to remove from the diet because they are ubiquitous in our society. In addition, this diet can cause a yo-yo effect because of the rapid weight loss that occurs during the first two weeks. Also, this diet can cause deficiencies, but also bring saturated lipids into the body because of the overconsumption of meat and fish. In fact, farmed meat does not have the same nutritional qualities as a game consumed in the Paleolithic era.

However, by consuming foods in accordance with our genetic heritage, we, therefore, lower the risk of getting seriously ill. It would, therefore, be sufficient to replace sugar, cereals, bread, and pasta with meat, fish, fruit, roots, vegetables, and nuts.

Chapter Five
Foods And Common Mistakes You Must Not Consider When On The Paleo Diet

Did you start the paleo diet but you still don't feel as good as you would like? Are you struggling to digest? Not resting well and enough?

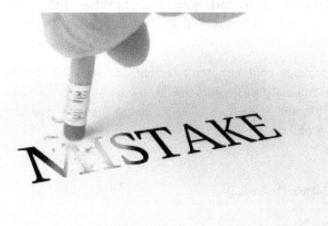

The following are Foods and Common Mistakes You Must not consider When on the Paleo Diet:

CONSUMING TOO MUCH FRUIT BECAUSE IT IS NATURAL FOOD

When we adopt a new diet that we consider healthy, many of us make the mistake of replacing junk food with industrial quantities of fruit, juices, and juices every hour of the day. The fact that fruit grows on trees does not mean that eating it continuously is always a good idea.

The fruit is more or less rich in fructose, which in large quantities causes inflammation, insulin response, and fat accumulation. Obviously, we are not talking about moderate amounts of low glycemic index fruit at meals or as snacks in active and metabolically healthy people. But for all the others, it is good to remember that the fruit contains sugar. And as such it should be handled with care.

BELIEVING THAT FRUIT JUICES ARE HEALTHY

Fruit juices are often perceived as healthy, maybe it's because they come from fruit, right? Well, not always. Often (to be optimistic) commercial fruit juices are added with sugars and sweeteners of all kinds. It may also be that the juice does not contain any fruit, but only water, sugar, and some chemical fruit smelling concoction. But even if you can drink 100% real juices, you shouldn't drink juice (or at least not so much). The whole fruit contains some sugar, but it is linked to fiber, which slows the release of sugar in the blood. While fruit juice is different. It contains no fiber, no resistance to chewing and nothing to prevent us from swallowing massive amounts of sugar in a few seconds.

A cup of orange juice contains about two orange sugar. And the sugar contained in commercial juices is very similar to sugary drinks like Coca-Cola. So, eat whole fruit, and avoid fruit juices if you are trying to lose weight or have metabolic problems.

HOPE TO LOSE 20 KG. IN A WEEK

Seeing people feeling disappointed who after a week of paleo diet didn't lose enough weight. Of course, you will need to be patient. Since there is no healthy and sustainable diet in the world, in the long run, you lose all the extra pounds in weeks. For that, do the minestrone diet. But then, after a few weeks, you will have a hunger crisis and eat the whole fridge.

INCREASE WITH THE CONSUMPTION OF SEEDS AND NUTS

Nuts and seeds are absolutely part of the paleo diet. But they are rich in calories and above all contain quantities of polyunsaturated fats. In particular, omega-6, of which we are already quite supplied by consuming products of animal origin. Especially if these products come from animals raised in an unethical way and fed with soy and cereals.

The other problem is the anti-nutrients contained in these foods. Specifically, phytic acid. This substance is found in most plants, especially in the shell of the wheat, in the nuts and the seeds. It acts as a protection against insects, birds and other external agents. And although it is digested by cows and sheep, it is not digestible for humans.

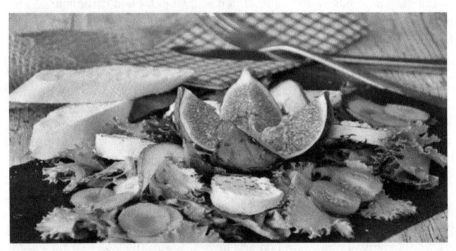

Phytic acid binds to minerals (especially iron and zinc) in foods, preventing their absorption. It also interferes with the enzymes needed to digest food, such as pepsin (protein), amylase (starch) and trypsin (proteins in the small intestine). There is no official indication, but it appears that an amount between 100 to 400 mg per day is tolerable. To get an idea, 100 grams of almonds contain 1300 mg of phytic acid. However, there is a fairly simple way to reduce phytic acid in nuts and seeds.

AFRAID OF FAT

It is not surprising that after decades of propaganda, many people are still afraid of fat. Despite the deepening and understanding of the paleo principles, when we talk about fats, many people are still wary and take fat off the meat or cook as little oil as possible. Often with disastrous results, and with low-calorie diets, low in fat and carbohydrates. Then maybe they develop hypothyroidism and take it with the Paleolithic diet.

THINK THAT FATTY FOODS MAKE YOU FAT

It seems intuitive to deduce that eating fat makes you fat. For the simple fact that the thing that collects under the skin and that makes us look soft and chubby is called fat. So eating fat should make us even fatter. But it's not that simple. Although 1 gram of fat has more calories than 1 gram of carbohydrates or protein, high-fat diets don't make people fat. And as with all things, it depends on the context. A diet high in fat and carbohydrates at the same time will make you fat, but not because of fat. In fact, diets rich in fat (and low in carbohydrates) cause a greater loss of fat than diets that are low in fat

BELIEVING THAT SATURATED FATS HURT

Some tens of years ago it was decided that the heart disease epidemic was caused by the consumption of too much fat, and in particular, by saturated fat. This decision was based on studies and political choices, today considered and proven to be completely wrong.

An impressive review published in 2010 that considered 21 epidemiological studies with a total of 347,747 subjects led to the following results: no association between saturated fat and heart disease. The idea that saturated fats increased the risk of heart attack is an unproven theory that somehow became a popular belief.

While it is established that consuming saturated fats increases the amount of HDL (good cholesterol) in the blood and changes the consistency of LDL cholesterol particles, from small and dense (dangerous) to large and soft (harmless).

CONSUMING THE EGG WHITE AND THROW THE EGG YOLK

There is one thing that most nutritionists do with great success: demonizing incredibly healthy foods. The suspected number one are the eggs, which containing amounts of cholesterol are considered responsible for the increased risk of heart disease. But recently it has been proven that cholesterol in the diet does not increase blood cholesterol. In fact, eggs primarily increase good cholesterol and are not associated with an increase in heart disease.

What remains is that eggs are one of the most nutritious foods that exist in nature. They are rich (especially the yolk) in every type of nutrient together with unique antioxidants that protect our eyes.

DON'T CONSUME ENOUGH CALORIES

When you eat real food, calories are a direct marker of nutrition. If you consume more calories from healthy food, it is wise to assume that you are also getting more nutrients. If you suffer from adrenal or thyroid problems, it may be more difficult to stabilize your blood sugar with fewer calories. Studies show that a low-calorie diet can cause a decrease in thyroid function or that it reduces its production of thyroid hormones.

To have a healthy metabolism, you need to make sure that you are consuming enough calories for your metabolic needs. This is mainly important for people who have already been diagnosed with adrenal and thyroid conditions. Low-calorie diets can also lead to hypoglycemia which can cause cortisol and insulin spikes.

TRYING TO PREPARE ANY DISH IN PALEO SAUCE

When you meet new vegetarians, they are usually interested in finding meat substitute foods for all the foods they abandoned with the new diet. So they consume hot dogs, sausages and other industrialized and often quite disgusting foods.

And the same thing happens to many Paleo diet newbies. They try to Paleolithic any food. This does not mean that we cannot occasionally give ourselves some paleo muffins, but as long as it does not become the rule in our diet.

Although these same contain paleo ingredients, they can contribute significantly to glycemic peaks or accentuate certain problems, especially in the presence of autoimmune conditions, bearing in mind that very often, in these recipes are considered large quantities of foods like nuts, seeds, and eggs. All foods that do not get along with autoimmune diseases and gastrointestinal problems.

IGNORING THE NUMBER OF PORTIONS

Despite what people say, calories do matter. And it is not true that by following the paleo diet you can eat when and how much you want. Especially if you are overweight and intend to lose weight. The inability to lose weight depends on various factors, but one of them certainly depends on the foods you choose. And for simplicity, especially when you are hungry and in a hurry, nuts and fruit seem to be the perfect combination. Maybe with a tablespoon of coconut butter. Let me be clear, these are perfectly paleo foods, but to be used with care and according to the objectives.

EAT LOTS OF SMALL MEALS DURING THE DAY

The idea that you have to eat so many small meals throughout the day to keep your metabolism active is a myth that makes no sense. It is true that eating increases the metabolism slightly during the digestive phase, but it is the total amount of food that determines the energy used, and not the number of meals.

Controlled studies where a group consumed many small meals and another group the same amount of food in fewer meals show that there is no difference between the two groups. In fact, a study conducted on obese subjects revealed that consuming 6 meals a day caused less sensation of satiety compared to 3 meals a day.

Not only is eating often useless in most people, but it can also be counterproductive. It is not natural for the human body to be continuously in a state of nourishment. Our ancestors used to fast from time to time and certainly did not eat the amount of food we consume today (in addition to quality, of course). When we do not eat for a prolonged period, a cellular process called autophagy cleans up the waste products from our cells.

Therefore, there is no evidence to show that consuming many small meals during the day is better than a few and more abundant meals. Not eating from time to time is good. If you have adrenal or glycemic problems, that's another story. And fasting is not for you then.

DO NOT EXPOSE YOURSELF TO THE SUN

Week after week, studies that confirm the importance of vitamin D increase. Despite this, many people avoid getting exposed to the sun and are covered with sunscreen for the sole pronunciation of the word sun. Why?

DO NOT COOK

It is impossible to follow the paleo diet without cooking. By doing so, you will not get results, and you will tire very soon. We are not talking about who knows what preparations. But if you plan to do your shopping once in a while and don't devote yourself to preparing your dishes, you'll flop.

We are talking about very simple things, like making a salad, cooking meat, fish and eggs and choosing fruit. And if you've been a world champion in pizza slices, restaurants, and frozen foods, you'll need a lot of discipline in the beginning. But your efforts will be amply repaid in all respects.

DO NOT DO PHYSICAL ACTIVITY

Sport is an important part of the Paleo style. If nutrition is a fundamental part, the importance of being physically active and lifting heavy loads from time to time should not be ignored. Paleo is not just a diet.

AVOID CARBOHYDRATES AT ALL COSTS AND FOR NO REASON

Many people who start paleo are attracted by the idea of losing weight fast while following a low-carb diet based on steak, eggs, avocado and coconut oil. If a low-carbohydrate diet can have therapeutic effects in some people, such as those with significant digestive problems, diabetes or diseases affecting cognitive function, there are many people who unnecessarily follow a low-carb or ketogenic paleo for the simple fact that they have been led to believe that nobody needs carbohydrates and that eating them will lead to disastrous health conditions. Many of these people are quite active, with intense workouts almost every day of the week. And this is not a good idea.

A perfect rule is not there, but if you are fickle, in perpetual lethargy, you are gaining weight despite the paleo, and you do not feel good as you would like with a paleo low-carb diet, you may find refreshment by increasing your carbohydrate consumption and improving your diet. Symptoms that you developed following an excessively low-carb diet.

EATING THE WRONG VEGETABLES

This recommendation is aimed primarily at people who have adopted a paleo diet due to digestive problems. For many people, paleo nutrition produces excellent digestive results. Eliminating cereals, dairy products and legumes can in many cases be enough to restore proper digestive function. But not for everyone. And some people, despite the paleo, don't solve their problems. Or even worse with paleo. Why? You may not be consuming enough carbohydrates to stimulate bowel movements. This could be due to a reduction in bowel function or the loss of healthy bacteria in the intestine (parasites). Or, especially in the presence of inflammatory diseases affecting the intestine, perhaps you are eating too many vegetables. The wrong kind. In particular, those vegetables rich in nature.

That is some types of carbohydrates that can feed certain classes of bacteria. In a healthy person, this is an absolutely positive thing. We feed healthy bacteria and protect ourselves from infections. In people with intestinal problems, it is possible that we are in the presence of an overgrowth of pathogenic bacteria. If this is the case, consuming universally healthy foods like apples and Brussels sprouts can create considerable stress and make us feel like a rag.

THINKING THAT BEING THIN IS EQUIVALENT TO BEING HEALTHY

Although it is always better not to be overweight, to be thin or to look fit does not mean that everything works perfectly inside. It is absolutely possible to be thin and diabetic. Being thin and getting a heart attack. Being thin and getting sick of any other disease. The external image is not everything. But not even remotely. This is a cultural, often disastrous illusion.

USE SUPPLEMENTS TO REMEDY BAD HABITS

Remember that companies that produce vitamins and supplements are also profit-oriented entities. Many people like to believe they can eat any crap, remedying this bad habit with some supplement. There is no such thing. Supplements are only supplements. They can be a powerful and very useful addition to a healthy diet, but they can never be a substitute for a healthy diet.

BELIEVING OUR DESTINY IS ALREADY WRITTEN IN OUR GENES

Even by the standards of the most conservative geneticists, we have control of our genetic expression between 80 and 97%. We all have dormant genes for anything, good or bad. You are not fat because your mother and father were fat. Nor are you destined to have a heart attack just because half of the people in your family have had one. And so on for diabetes, multiple sclerosis, and other diseases.

Genetics can certainly have some influence, but genes are turned on and off by regulatory genes, and regulatory genes are controlled primarily by nutrients. A gene will not express itself unless the internal environment favors its expression. And we have maximum control over this through the foods we eat, the emotions we experience, the toxicity of the environment in which we live and the lifestyle we choose to follow.

THINKING THAT A VEGAN DIET IS MORE "NATURAL"

All of us, regardless of our ideologies, ethnicity or religion, are genetically hunter-gatherers and 99.99% identical to our ancestors lived from 40,000 to 100,000 years ago. We are, in effect, creatures of the ice age, designed to consume a diet rich in foods of animal origin and natural fats, along with a variety of vegetable fiber.

Vegetarianism and veganism are modern ideas based more on ideological principles than on principles of human physiology and anthropological evidence.

Foods from animal sources are as healthy as their source, and no one should eat meat from animals raised in an unethical way, fed on cereals and forced to undergo hormonal treatments and antibiotics.

The alternative is not to be vegetarian or vegan. The alternative is to find foods derived from healthily raised animals. Plant foods are excellent, and a source of many antioxidants and phytonutrients, needed today more than ever. But these alone are far from being all we need to live healthily.

BELIEVING THAT FOLLOWING, THE PALEO DIET IS TOO EXPENSIVE

Nothing is further from reality. With a little organization, you can save money compared to a "normal" diet. Not to mention the money we will eventually save to go to the doctor when we are very "big."

GIVING IN TO THE IDEA OF EVERYTHING OR NOTHING

The typical worry of those who start paleo: can I do paleo diet even if I have a tight budget and can't afford grass-fed meat, organic vegetables and fruits?

The short answer is: yes.

And the mistake many newcomers make is to abandon the paleo because their budget does not allow them to always choose the best option. In case, if choosing the best products is not always possible, here are some practical tips:

1. if you buy non-grass-fed meat, choose lean cuts. And it eliminates the visible fat before cooking.
2. if you can buy organic vegetables and fruits, choose the one you would eat with peel (apples instead of oranges, for example).
3. Limit paleo sweets that often require the use of rather expensive flours.

BUNCHING ON LOW-FAT AND LOW-CARB PROTEIN

Reviewing your diet often matches the reduction of carbohydrate consumption (these vary from person to person). What often happens is that people who choose to follow a low-carb regime do not eat enough fat, filling their plates with protein foods. So you often end up eating salads with a teaspoon of olive oil and unheard of chicken. This is the classic way to hurt yourself.

In the end, we are consuming a low-carb and even low-fat, but excessively high in protein diet. For those who choose a low-carb approach, it is appropriate to increase fat consumption and reduce protein consumption, with more or less reduced amounts of carbohydrates (depending on the objectives and physical activity).

ELIMINATE GLUTEN BUT EAT GLUTEN-FREE PACKAGED FOODS

You have decided to abandon the cereals, but then you have chosen a gluten-free diet. Excellent decision, but eating gluten-free bread is not ideal. Most (not to say all) of gluten-free sandwiches, pizzas, and desserts undergo major industrial changes and contain very low-quality vegetable oils (always to be avoided) and preservatives. In addition to having a noticeable glycemic impact, which is not what we hope for in most cases with a paleo diet.

REPLACE BARREL SUGAR WITH HONEY AND AGAVE JUICE

You have decided to eliminate the sugar, but the desire for sugar has not yet gone. So switch to "healthy" sweeteners like honey and agave juice. Agave is based on fructose and will not make you a nice long-term service. Honey, which contains less fructose than agave juice, should be used sparingly. Especially if you're trying to lose weight. The best alternative is to resist, integrating with a bit of glutamine and eventually, use a little stevia, waiting for the adaptation step to pass and your body learns to use the new fuel at its best.

ASK YOURSELF ANY PALEO QUESTION

There are people who want to see whatever happens in their lives through the Paleolithic lens. Computers and modern medicine did not exist in the Paleolithic era. So, shouldn't we use them? It could also be so, but we have the benefit of modern science and research to combine with the paleo diet, to get the best possible results, and it would be unreasonable not to make use of the opportunity.

DON'T LEAVE YOUR BODY TIME TO ADAPT

Sometimes the body needs some time, especially if you are experiencing chronic discomfort. Take all the time you need.

ABANDON THE DIET BECAUSE YOU ARE LOSING TOO MUCH WEIGHT

Did you start the paleo diet and you were skinny? And are you continuing to lose weight? So you decide to go back to old habits. It happens, but there could be a problem like an excess of intestinal permeability with relative malabsorption. Or you are simply not eating enough. Consume a lot, and maybe you do intense physical activity. You can increase the amount of fat. Or carbohydrates like fruit. Or add starches like potatoes.

CHECK CONTINUOUSLY

It is important to be aware of your state of health. A person who is well, will not notice particular variations in his well-being, but in the presence of pathological conditions such as inflammatory or autoimmune diseases, the speech changes. And even a single piece of bread or a glass of milk could restart the inflammatory process and bring you back to a state of chaos. So if you resist early on, it is very likely that you will no longer have any remorse or desire to consume old foods.

BELIEVING THAT THE PALEO DIET IS JUST A DIET

Paleo is a holistic lifestyle that includes nutrition but also other factors such as exercise, sleep and stress management. If you cannot recognize sleep as a key component of your health, you are forgetting an essential ingredient. Sleep assists you in the regulation of weight, stress, hormones, and metabolism.

NOT SLEEPING WELL AND ENOUGH

Sleeping is an essential part of a healthy lifestyle, and it is probably the most important factor. Without adequate sleep, you can follow a perfect paleo diet along with a fitness regimen, but you will never achieve the best shape. Without getting 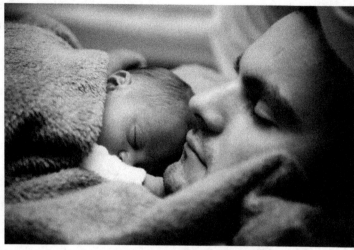 enough sleep, your body does not work properly, it does not fully recover after physical activity, and you find it difficult to keep stress under control. Finding out why you are not sleeping like you should and trying to understand the reasons and solve them is a necessary step to improve your health.

CONSUME FOODS TOO RICH OF AGES

AGEs stand for Advanced glycation end-products. That is compounds that are naturally formed in the body by the chemical reaction between sugars and proteins. If the concentration of AGEs in the blood becomes excessive, these final products can cause damage to almost any tissue and organ in our body. In practice, they act to permanently activate low-grade inflammation by binding to cellular receptors known as RAGEs. These reactions, when excessive, appear to be associated with premature aging and most chronic diseases such as type 2 diabetes, Alzheimer's, autoimmune diseases, etc.

The good news is that for those who follow the Paleo diet, most of these problems are reduced. Fruits and vegetables, as well as eggs, are poor in AGEs. And also raw meat and fish. But it's not like we can always eat meat.

It is in fact when we cook meat and fish, which increases the formation of AGEs. And the worst way to do it is by cooking at high temperatures (embers, barbecues). Therefore, it is preferable to choose gentler cooking methods such as using the slow cooker, which minimizes the number of AGEs but still guarantees adequate cooking and gourmet flavors.

Chapter Six
Amazing ways to Incorporate the Paleo Diet into Your Lifestyle

If you've ever looked around for a diet program to help you lose a few inches, you've probably come across the Paleo diet. At first glance, it doesn't seem to be much about the Paleo diet, very popular, and low in carbohydrates, high in protein, and free of processed foods.

Making the transition from today's diet to that of our ancestors is not necessarily easy. Depending on what you expect from the paleo diet, your life situation and your ultimate goal (to stay in the paleo or not), you may have the interest to go gradually according to the Japanese method of small steps. We present here three gradual stages of the paleo diet, which can be adapted one after the other, depending on what you want.

It is, in short, a diet that eliminates all foods that have appeared since the Neolithic with the advent of agriculture (salt, sugar, dairy products, cereals, legumes but also refined oils). Why? Because if our DNA has remained the same since the Paleolithic, our diet has changed radically from that time and much more since the industrial revolution. The food that we are adapted to, that which allows us to be the fittest and healthy, would be that of the Paleolithic: fresh food from hunting or gathering (meat, fish, poultry, eggs, vegetables and fruits, nuts and seeds, herbs and spices). Exit the baguette, lentils, cheese and all industrial foods.

It's a no-brainer that our caveman ancestors don't have a lot of food choices back in the day. As such, you are only allowed to feed on grass meat, fish, fruit, vegetables, eggs, nuts and seeds, and some oils (olive, nuts, flax seeds, macadamia nuts, avocado, coconut).

This means that things like cereals, legumes, refined sugar, dairy products, refined vegetable oils, processed foods, and even salt are off-limits. It is rare, however, to eat three non-Paleo meals a week. So in theory, you should be able to indulge in the occasional beer or slice of pizza, right?

By eating what corresponds to the original functions of the organism, it is indeed reduced, but one could also prevent a number of diseases, especially those called civilization. Changing your diet is not easy. It is necessary, even for the most motivated ones, to face temporary discomfort and to unlearn food. That's why the specialists of this diet now propose to gradually follow the example of dietitian-nutritionist.

We will now offer you three progressive stages to move to the paleo, each in their way you will already do good. Sure you can go directly to the 3rd stage without passing through the square.

Step 1: The Basic Paleo

Aim: eliminate industrial foods, better choose others, say goodbye to gluten

At this point, it's all about better choosing your food. The big restriction is no longer eating gluten. Why start with him? Because a priori is the elimination of gluten that has the most beneficial effect on health. For bread, if you used to eat baguette or white bread and you cannot imagine life without, you can introduce an extra step of replacing your white bread with a whole loaf of bread or leavened cereals. And by decreasing as much as possible your portions.

Foods to avoid

- Cakes, buns, and pastries
- Industrial foods containing additives
- Alcoholic drinks containing gluten and sugar (beer, cocktails)
- Grain products (bread, pasta, biscuits)
- Legumes (soy, lentils, dried beans)
- Sugar and sweets

Authorized foods

- Meat, eggs, fish and other foods high in animal protein
- Good fats (olive oil, coconut oil, animal fat, avocado, butter)
- Vegetables, fruits, nuts, hazelnuts, almonds
- Herbs and spices
- Dairy products
- Dark chocolate with more than 70% cocoa, honey

- Tea, coffee without sugar

You usually eat Bread, Treats and industrial snacks, Sugar, legumes, Cereals with gluten (pasta, semolina, wheat, etc.), Sunflower oil,

Replace it with Paleo bread, buckwheat in all its forms, Chocolate with 90% cocoa, nuts, and raw seeds, Honey, Vegetables (sweet potato for example), Cereals without gluten (rice, quinoa, millet, buckwheat), Olive or coconut oil.

Step 2: The Classic Paleo

Aim: those of the basic paleo + end of dairy products and cereal products (even without gluten)

If you have not done it yet, it's time to say goodbye to bread. And also cheese, yogurt, and milk. For butter, it is possible to clarify it to extract lactose. Some Paleo authors maintain it at this stage arguing that it contains little lactose anyway.

Foods to avoid

- Cakes, buns, and pastries
- Industrial foods containing additives
- Alcoholic drinks containing gluten and sugar (beer, cocktails)
- Grain products (bread, pasta, biscuits)
- Legumes (soy, lentils, dried beans)
- Sugar and sweets
- Dairy products

Authorized foods

- Meat, eggs, fish and other foods high in animal protein
- Good fats (olive oil, coconut oil, animal fat, avocado, clarified butter)
- Vegetables, fruits, nuts, hazelnuts, almonds
- Herbs and spices
- Dark chocolate with more than 70% cocoa, honey
- Tea, coffee without sugar (but in limited quantity)

You usually eat Bread, Treats and industrial snacks, Sugar, legumes, Cereals, Sunflower oil, Tea and coffee, Milk.

Replace it with Paleo bread, Chocolate with 90% cocoa, nuts, and raw seeds, Honey, Vegetables (sweet potato for example), Nuts, natural seeds, Olive or coconut oil, Herbal tea, Coconut milk,

Aim: those of the classic paleo + elimination of alcohol, tea, coffee, and chocolate

At this point, you will only eat food from the supermarket's fresh aisle (or better, bought directly from farmers from the market). It is about consuming the most "raw" foods possible. More alcohol, more tea, coffee, chocolate. On the social level, it's more restrictive. This may require you to have your food at hand if you are invited.

If you are at this stage, it is most often because of strong personal conviction (ecological for example) or because of health disorders you have led there.

Foods to avoid

- Cakes, buns, and pastries
- Industrial foods
- Grain products (bread, pasta, biscuits)
- Legumes (soy, lentils, dried beans)
- Sugar and sweets
- Dairy products
- All alcohols
- Tea, coffee, dark chocolate

Authorized foods

- Meat, eggs, fish and other foods high in animal protein
- Good fats (olive oil, coconut oil, animal fat, avocado, clarified butter)
- Vegetables, fruits, nuts, hazelnuts, almonds
- Herbs and spices

You usually eat Bread, Treats and industrial snacks, Sugar, legumes, Cereals, Sunflower oil, Tea and coffee, Milk, Alcohol, Chocolate.

Replace it with Paleo bread, Chocolate with 90% cocoa, nuts, and raw seeds, Honey, Vegetables (sweet potato for example), Nuts, natural seeds, Olive or coconut oil, Herbal tea, Coconut milk, Water, Coconut Chips.

In any case, whatever the stage, to follow a paleo diet in the world today, it is better to keep in mind to eat Paleo 80% of your time and give yourself a 20% margin for outings, and invitations.

Chapter Seven
Time to Prepare Your Kitchen for the Paleo Diet

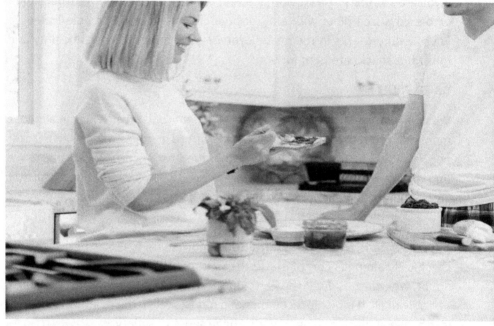

Preparing healthy and nutritious Paleo diet snacks in your kitchen is easier than it seems. Often we tend to consider the moment of the snack as a bad food habit, but in reality, it is we who do not know how to make good use of it. In fact, due to a bad food organization, most people (especially in the late afternoon, in work or study places) take refuge behind the display of a "junk food machine"; in the throes of hunger attacks.

Certainly, this does not mean to have a snack! At least not that healthy and dietetic snack contemplated by the Paleo diet. In all those cases it is obvious that this is not a good food habit. So the physiological problems will begin to be felt chronically, at least as chronic as the intake of these junk foods without nutrients and that affect human health.

Being able to choose, in these cases, it is preferable to avoid having a snack.

If you are also of this opinion but you are not going to go hungry, then this is for you! You'll find lots of interesting ideas to make your Paleo Snacks to take wherever and whenever you want. Easy to make and practical to carry, Paleo Snack fits perfectly with an authentic and natural lifestyle. It doesn't matter if you are a young girl, a student, a career woman, a family man or a pensioner who enjoys free time: with a bit of organization, you will be able to realize your healthy snacks in the hectic everyday life. Find out which healthy and nutritious snacks are right for you:

DRIED FRUIT MIX

Versatile and practical, dried fruit is an excellent food for snacking in all those moments and those days where you can't afford anything more than a jacket pocket. A real health pocket; in fact, the dried fruit is rich in cerebral active nutrients that improve general cognitive functions. A handful of dried fruit gives strength and energy precisely in those hours where fatigue begins to be felt.

If we now consider that dried fruit does not create halitosis problems and specifically almonds contribute to the natural whitening of teeth, without a doubt, we can consider it the Paleo Snack idea that is the smartest and most versatile of all. It is highly recommended not to overdo the quantities; the risk is to arrive at lunch or dinner, with a huge sense of satiety.

BOILED EGGS

A hard-boiled egg that is eaten in 2 bites.

Why not? Eggs are not only a fundamental ingredient for seasoning and filling a recipe, but they are also an excellent snack (practical and healthy) that can be enjoyed in the hectic everyday life. In reality, it is a question of having a bit of organization in the morning. Pause 30 seconds in the kitchen to boil the eggs before entering the shower, and you're done.

10 minutes later (for example the shower time) drain the boiled eggs and let them cool before placing them in the Tupperware. Furthermore, the eggs have a high level of conservation, and the shell protects them from any external contamination.

Let the eggs cool naturally and keep them in the fridge for a week if possible:

- You will have to remember to prepare your snack eggs 1, maximum 2 times a week.
- So the real difficulty lies in being able to consolidate new eating habits! Because otherwise an egg is eaten in 2 bites and its benefits are lasting.
- Such a high level of protein (as many as 7 g) in so little food.

Furthermore, egg proteins are vital because they contain essential amino acids and all in usable form; that is, those that the human body cannot produce on its own in a manner sufficient to satisfy the physical needs:

- Phenylalanine;
- isoleucine;
- Lysine;
- Leucine;
- Methionine;
- threonine;
- Tryptophan;
- Valine.

Eggs are considered by the medicine an essential food for pregnant women and during the lactation period:

The high level of choline (or Vitamin J, an essential coenzyme for the constitution of cell membranes) present in eggs, contributes to the healthy and rigorous development of the nervous system of the fetus and prevents it from congenital diseases.

Essential, natural, practical and long-lasting; boiled eggs are an excellent healthy snack, to be taken into consideration among the Paleo Snack ideas that can be enjoyed in the hectic everyday life.

WILD BERRY VARIETY

The colors of the forest in practical takeaway trays.

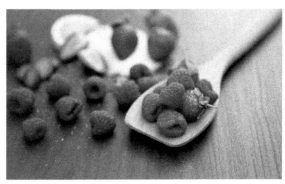

Fresh, colorful and of a thousand varieties the fruits of the undergrowth (precisely because they share their habitat despite having properties and distinctive characteristics between them) have invaded our food. Just stop in the nearest shop in the city to fill a bag of berries, to be enjoyed in peace during the workday; when hunger begins to strike.

In fact, berries (all fruit in general) is always recommended to take it away from meals in order to be able to synthesize as many vitamins (nutrients) as possible quickly, precisely when the intestine is not processing other foods. Excellent as essential to take out of meals; wild berries are a sweet healthy snack, to be taken into consideration among the Paleo Snack ideas that can be enjoyed in the hectic everyday life.

BANANA & APPLE

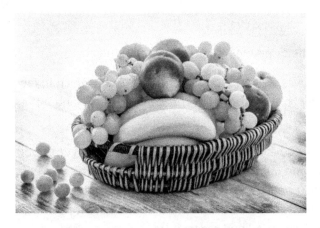

The choice is yours; apple or banana?

Banana and apple are the perfect combinations to alternate as an everyday snack. When the preparation gets out of hand, you can always look back and pick up an apple, or turn sideways and rip a banana out of its helmet.

"One day, apple, one day, banana ... you live for 100 years!"

DATES & PRUNES FROM CALIFORNIA

With dark color and a unique flavor: California plums.

Dried because it is dehydrated (i.e., released from all liquids) the California Plum and rich in nutrients, a true elixir of well-being. Already packaged, easy to find and with good preservation, the California plums and dried dates in effect acquire a place among the most comfortable and common Paleo Snack ideas to find. Real healthy snacks that reduce the sense of fatigue contribute to the health and shine of skin and hair.

Also California plums:

- they are very rich in copper, potassium, magnesium, vitamin B6 and K;
- contribute to the normal functioning of the digestive system;
- they regulate and maintain the level of cholesterol in the blood.

Superfoods! Go easy on the greed! Especially if you are on a Paleo diet. Dried fruit contains a medium or high GI (Glycemic Index)

THE DRIED MEAT

Fine meat rich in history. The dried meat fine as per tradition.

Nothing to do with other over-the-counter gourmet products, which in fact often contain carcinogenic preservatives (Nitrite and Nitrate) and other additives.

With rather modest origins, the dried meat has then conquered the food market as a niche product and quite delicious. In fact, originally the best cuts were intended for the consumption of fresh meat, while the less tender parts of the meat and the particularly adult meats were seasoned with salt and other spices (therefore: salted, dried and seasoned).

The main purpose of the poor people was to be able to satisfy the demand for meat all year round, and drying the meat was the only solution.

But when the needs of people are transformed into traditions, delicious techniques, short chain processes; the dried meat has known its true fame.

AVOCADO STUFFED WITH GUACAMOLE; INGENIOUS INVENTION

It takes no more than 10 minutes of preparation (just peel the avocado and crush it with lemon, oil, salt, pepper, and coriander). You can pour the cream into a small takeaway jar (airtight), which is then placed inside a larger Tupperware, so as to carry two carrots, a cucumber, and a knife to peel the vegetables in a single container.

The benefits of avocado are innumerable, in fact, rich in potassium and calcium; it is an essential food to maintain the health of the skin, hair, and brain. In addition, the avocado contains significant amounts of monounsaturated fats that prevent the risk of diabetes and defend the heart from cardiovascular diseases.

A, B1, B2, D, E, K, H, and PP are the innumerable vitamins present in a single fruit.

Maybe it doesn't represent the maximum in terms of practicality, but anyone in the nutrition world (Paleo or not Paleo) would recommend a nice pudding of avocado for a snack.

SELECTION OF OLIVES

Simple Olives, what could be more natural and authentic than making a snack by munching on so-called healthy fats? Olives certainly deserve a place among the Paleo Snack ideas that can be enjoyed in the hectic everyday life, even if the strong stimulating effect of the appetite must be pointed out.

Make sure you have at least 2 or 3 nuts in your drawer if you don't want to risk sinking your teeth into the desk from hunger.

CRUSHED ALMOND

Homemade organic almond crushed.

A puree with an explosive and enthralling taste, you won't be able to stop. To be jealously guarded in the secret drawer of our office, ready to pop out at the first event. Excellent accompanied with fruit; with the weighing of almonds, it is easy to transform a simple banana into a delicious Paleo Snack, which can be enjoyed as a snack in the hectic everyday life.

Almond cream is completely natural, with no added colorings, additives or palm oil. Not only is it not harmful to health but it also contains all the healthy properties of almond concentrated in an explosion of taste.

CRISPY ALGAE

Fine and crunchy algae, the favorite snack of the Japanese.

If you are a lover of sushi and oriental cuisine, your diet can only include an excellent and healthy snack based on crispy algae. Spreadable and toasted are a valid alternative to crackers and chips; with the incomparable difference that (in addition to not being harmful) algae act as a healthy remedy for various psychosomatic problems.

Rich in:

- minerals,
- vitamins (A, B, C, E, and K),
- fibers;

- and in view of the great practicality in transport and consumption, crispy algae deserve a place among the Paleo Snack ideas, usable in the hectic everyday life.

A HANDFUL OF SEEDS

Pocket and smart as the gesture of pulling the crumbs to the pigeons the seeds of:

- pumpkin,
- poppy,
- sunflower,
- sesame,
- linen,
- they are an excellent natural hunger break with a very high nutritional value.

The seed mix is a classic among the Paleo Snack ideas to propose in any circumstance.

ORGANIC COCONUT DRINK

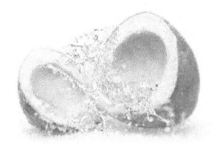

Pure coconut water directly from the fruit. Rich in fiber, enzymes, magnesium, and potassium, it also has the advantage of being naturally sweet (with no added sugar). It is said to be one of the beauty secrets of the great world stars. If you feel like a superstar, all you have to do is follow the wave of success and start sipping the elixir of youth too.

Superstars aside, the coconut organic drink is a great Paleo Snack idea to sip in the hectic everyday life.

Chapter Eight
Paleo Diet for Families with Kids

The philosophy of the Paleolithic diet is that the ideal diet corresponds to that of our ancestors. One of the greatest determinants of our nutritional needs is our genes. And since our genes have not changed (0.02%), that's why we should eat like our ancestors. The paleo diet, also known as the ancestral diet, therefore focuses on a diet low in carbohydrates but high in fiber and protein. Lean meats, poultry, fish and seafood, eggs, nuts and seeds, and low-starch fruits and vegetables (i.e., no potatoes, yams, etc.) are preferred. However, this diet excludes dairy products, grain products, legumes and salted or processed foods (canned goods, cakes, soft drinks, etc.).

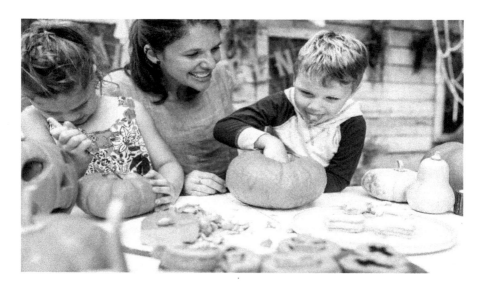

Nutrition in children and even more so nutrition education in children touches them because as a parent who has little kids, and you daily try to teach them what are the real foods, those of nature, and to consciously choose what to eat.

The problem of nutrition in children peeps out among new parents shortly after the birth of their young. In fact, after 5/6 months from birth, some pediatricians propose weaning and the insertion of the first baby food. Even if the nutrition of our children is correct, it begins even before birth, because they absorb the nutrients and anti-nutrients that mothers ingest, so we must think about eating at best even during the period of pregnancy.

Observing the rules of the Paleo diet in a family with children is quite easy until one is confronted with the outside world, therefore with the nursery school, the kindergarten, the birthday parties of the friends but also simply the gardens. In these places, your children will see other children eating things "different" from theirs. In your eyes they are junk, to them, they are something they have never seen, tasted, and surely they are intrigued.

For this reason, it is important to teach people to choose consciously and not feel obligated to make a choice because they said, mom and dad. This of course if there are no serious allergies or autoimmune diseases that require strict control of the food consumed by our children.

Some children at school eat exactly what other children eat (because some of them don't have any particular pathologies or allergies), but when some of them leave school they bring a fruit, or a paleo sweet, like paleo cookies or paleo muffins, and at breakfast and dinner instead they eat natural and unprocessed foods granted in the Paleo Diet. They are very fortunate because some of the school that these children attend is very attentive to food, to snack, centrifuges or extracts, and desserts are made daily and not packaged.

In any case, the best advice is to let your child taste everything, always at the clinical level, if possible, and make them choose what is good and what is not.

For example, that children easily realize the "damage" caused by "modern" food, another example is if they eat potato chips at a party, the next day or evening itself often has blisters in their mouth that burn them, or if they eat packaged ice cream the next day they have a blocked nose or another simple sign that we can teach them to recognize is the burning bottom. Children know very well that these little annoyances are due to what they ate and soon learn to adjust themselves.

The paleo diet is to feed only ingredients that our prehistoric ancestors had access. Meat, fish, fruits, vegetables, eggs, and nuts are at the heart of these recipes. This offers parents baby recipes based on this very special diet. According to doctors, this baby recipe contains ten times more vitamin A than the recommended daily intake for a toddler.

Today Paleo Diet is the right diet for families with kids, which can be very useful to mothers and fathers who always have little time. And then even being able to prepare dinner in no time can be very useful. The diet is a natural recipe for messy families and also enhance mental fitness for a kid, Paleo Diet aims to accompany families to discover a healthy, practical and enjoyable food style based on the prehistoric era.

In fact, how can a natural and healthy kitchen be combined with a family with limited time, in today's hectic life? This is the mission of " The Paleo Diet ", the diet for mothers and fathers with little time but with the desire to gather the family around a table to savor the taste of simple, healthy, and delicious recipes.

It also benefits the kids psychologically and gives parents the chance to show how to bring children closer to food and sheds light on some important aspects related to nutrition and health.

How to educate your children to an evolutionary diet?

As a parent you can personally follow the Paleo Diet when your kid is 1-year-old, so you can start the classic weaning following the rules dictated by the pediatrician, starting with the tapioca and vegetable broth, then introducing one vegetable at a time, then meat and fish. You may resort to homogenized glass only in cases of "emergency" such as long journeys or to prepare a meal on the fly at times of heavy workload.

Otherwise, you will have to always prepare the homogenized vegetables, meat, and fish, the vegetable and meat broth, obviously starting from the raw materials and not using nuts or preparations nor salt. It seems difficult and a great waste of time but with the assurance, you will need only a few minutes of effort to prepare large quantities of homogenized which you can keep in the freezer. In this way you can mix proteins and vegetables at will, always offering new tastes to the child and giving their palate and digestive system to new natural foods. Another factor not to be neglected in preparing homogenized at home is that as the baby grows, you can blend the preparation less and less and propose it to the baby so that he learns to chew properly and gradually.

However, on the subject of nutrition for families with children as a serene parent who does not force and does not oblige them to eat one thing rather than another. The best approach is teaching.

Chapter Nine
Paleo Diet: The Perfect Breakfast Ideas

Breakfast is one of the most important daily meals that should be consumed by the individual and never give up, because of its importance in strengthening the body and make it able to do his meals daily to the fullest. This meal is characterized by its ability to maintain the ideal weight of the individual; do not affect the weight in the case of a diet program, unlike lunch and dinner.

With its diet based exclusively on nature, the Paleo diet is ideal to benefit your body and lose weight. Here are all the keys to a successful Paleo breakfast.

The "Paleolithic" diet advocates a return to the diet of our ancestors, which has multiple health benefits. It consists of eating only a variety of fruits, vegetables, meats, eggs, and seeds, that is unprocessed foods. And recipes for feasting at breakfast time are not lacking.

If you like fruit, you will be able to indulge yourself with delicious meals with cottage cheese and berries or with tasty and crunchy fruit granola. To surprise your taste buds when you wake up, try our coconut pudding, chia seeds, and red berries. What a delight! And to hydrate you, you can sip succulent mango, apple, lemon, and honey smoothie.

If you're more of a foodie and savory, you should enjoy our paleo bread and our salty pistachio cookies. To fill up on protein, you can make an omelet with tomato or little eggs spinach casserole. Simple and really tasty recipes that only need a few ingredients.

The Paleo diet can also create ultra-gourmet recipes that will delight the taste buds as soon as you wake up. Paleo muffins made with applesauce and rice flour will suit the whole family. Bowl cake with oatmeal will allow you to refuel for the day. It is prepared in a jiffy, and you can decline it according to your tastes and your desires.

Paleo breakfast can be problematic for some people who go on a paleo diet. The paleo diet prohibits industrially manufactured foods. For example, you can eat red meat, but not processed meat.

Let's look at the foods that are allowed under a paleo diet: fruits, vegetables, meat, oils, and nuts. For each food category, you will find examples that you can include for your paleo breakfast.

Fruits

Fruits are prominent in the paleo breakfast. Want to lose weight? In this case, choose fruits low in sugar for breakfast. Examples of common low sugar fruits:

- grapes
- Watermelon
- blueberries
- raspberries

Vegetables

Vegetables are preferred for fruits. Indeed, vegetables are much lower in sugar. You can eat at will. On the other hand, do not eat fried vegetables. Although most people prefer fruit, vegetables are a good place for breakfast. Here are some vegetables that you can incorporate into your paleo breakfast.

- asparagus
- carrots
- spinach

Meat

People on a paleo diet are encouraged to focus on meat at breakfast. Proteins and lipids go hand in hand, and that goes for the Paleo breakfast. No other diet encourages the consumption of red meat at breakfast. Here are some types of meat that you can incorporate into a paleo breakfast.

- Chicken thighs
- Chicken breast
- Salmon
- Lamb

Oils

One might think that oils should be avoided as much as possible since they are very rich in fat. However, this is a mistake: it is mainly carbohydrates that make you fat. Oils and fats of natural origin are important for the body. Here are some oils you can add to your paleo breakfast to get more energy:

- Coconut oil
- Olive oil
- Avocado oil
- Macadamia nut oil

Nuts

Nuts are very good for health, but very caloric. Be especially careful with cashews. Peanuts are often considered nuts, wrongly. Better not to consume it. Here are some examples of nuts that will go well with a paleo breakfast.

- Almonds
- Hazelnut
- Pecan nuts
- Nuts

The paleo diet is a complex diet. It's about consuming what our ancestors ate. For most foods, this will not be a problem, but there are exceptions. In particular, you must not consume meat from animals that have been fed on cereals. Some foods are to be excluded because they did not exist in prehistoric times. These products do not fit the paleo way of life, and therefore have no place in the paleo breakfast. Here are some examples of foods to give up:

- Legumes - for example, black beans, and peanuts
- Cereals - for example, rye and brown rice
- Added sugar - for example, in cakes and sweets
- Almost all dairy products
- Vegetable oils - for example, rapeseed oil and soybean oil

Better a lot of fat than a lot of carbohydrates. Research has shown that it is better for you to consume a lot of fat than a lot of carbohydrates. Participants in one study were divided into two groups. One group was on a high carbohydrate diet and the other group on a high-fat diet. As a result, the group whose diet was high in fat lost more weight. The high-fat diet has also led to a drop in blood pressure and low cholesterol. This study is proof of the power of the paleo diet.

The Standard Breakfast Is Far Too Rich in Carbohydrates

Often, the breakfast we eat is way too rich in carbohydrates. The fault lies not only with bread but also with cereals. A paleo breakfast excludes this type of food. To make it easier to switch to a paleo diet, it is important to have breakfast that you like. You do not want eggs or meat in the morning? No problem: there are many other solutions.

Ideas for A Perfect Paleo Breakfast

The difference between an ordinary dinner and a paleo dinner does not imply a drastic change. As part of the Paleo diet, the dinner poses a little problem when you think it is a diet. However, this is rarely the case with breakfast. Skip two slices of jam to a paleo breakfast is a big step. Here are some ideas to help you better appreciate your paleo breakfast.

1. Stop Counting Calories

With the paleo breakfast, no need to count the calories. Stick to the paleo recipes, and you'll lose weight fast. You can choose fruit depending on sugar content, but in principle, you do not have to think about how much you eat.

2. Try the bread or pancakes paleo

The paleo diet offers many possibilities to vary its diet, but sometimes we want food that we are familiar with. In this case, you can opt for paleo pancakes or make paleo bread, with all your favorite paleo ingredients. You can make crepes made from coconut milk, honey, and coconut flour. At first sight, making bread without cereals seems rather complicated, but there are dozens of delicious paleo bread recipes.

3. Prepare your breakfast the day before

Some bread from the bakery, a little butter, some jam and a glass of milk, and breakfast is ready! The paleo breakfast requires a little more effort. Accommodating the paleo diet in a busy life requires some changes. One idea is to prepare your dishes during the weekend, which you can easily warm up or take out of the freezer during the week. Paleo bread cooked on Sundays can provide breakfast for five days. You can even prepare your egg, meat and vegetable dishes the night before.

4. Do not be too strict about dairy

The consumption of dairy products is controversial. Our ancestors had no milking cows at their disposal. The other disadvantage of milk is that it is processed food. The benefits of milk for health are however proven. So do not be too strict and allow yourself to drink milk. It is better to opt for whole milk, which is less processed than skimmed milk and semi-skimmed milk.

▪ Nutrient Deficiency? Remove it

The Paleo diet has many health benefits, but between breakfast and two other meals of the day, it is possible to miss certain nutrients. Here are nutrients at risk of deficiency:

- Vitamin D
- Iodine (present in table salt)
- Magnesium
- Vitamin K2

You can solve this problem by adjusting your diet or taking supplements. Pay special attention to essential nutrients. It is better to observe the paleo diet with more flexibility than to risk one's health.

Chapter Ten
Day to Day Paleo Diet Recipes

The Paleolithic Diet is a diet that has been much talked about in recent years. It allows you to lose weight and keep the line without counting calories or eating less. But many criticize it, stressing that it can be dangerous to health.

It is based on a simple idea: we are programmed to be beautiful, strong and healthy. Our genes allow it. If we get fat, get sick and have little energy, the fault is what we eat. To have a sculpted physique, therefore, it would be enough to put on the table the foods that activate the "fat burning genes." What are these foods? Those who come from Prehistory!

Diseases unknown in antiquity, such as obesity, diabetes and celiac disease (gluten intolerance, a protein complex found in cereals), would, in fact, be born together with modern nutrition, which introduced dairy products and high-index carbohydrates into the diet glycemic. By eating as we used to do millions of years ago, we could lose weight, slow down aging, lower bad cholesterol and reduce appetite.

The paleo diet is an easy type of diet to follow because it does not include calorie counting. You can eat as much as you want and strengthen your muscles by losing weight. Just take an example from what our ancestors ate. For millions of years - before the advent of agriculture - the cave dwellers only ate meat, fish, fruit, and vegetables. Nothing too elaborate! If you want to follow this diet, you have to say goodbye to refined foods and flours like pasta, cereals, sweets and sweetened carbonated drinks and instead introduce olive or coconut oil and flax seeds! Like all diets. However, should be addressed in the correct way and before trying, it is advisable that you ask your family doctor for advice to understand if there may be contraindications.

The Paleo diet, also known as a digestive diet, focuses on food intake that a typical hunter's collection would have eaten. This means meat, eggs, fish, nuts, and algae, avoiding sugar, cereals and dairy products. Any diet plan involves inevitable boredom, a monotonous "same meal, different days" that makes the wagon easy to fall. But to keep you updated, we've developed a delicious seven-day meal plan - you can strictly follow it or just think about it.

Eggs, lean meat, vegetables, and nuts, which every self-respecting cave would have died, are ideal for eating healthy and offering an excellent alternative to processed foods such as cereals, salami, ready meals, and biscuits. The plan will help you lose weight, give you an extra protein stroke on a training day or give you a tasty recipe when you eat.

Monday

- Breakfast: Sausage Omelet (72 cal). Use coconut oil (826 cal) and 2-3 large eggs to cook (220 cal). Add two roasted turkey sausages (80 cal) and a handful of green vegetables (23 cal).
- Snack: Full of almonds (576 cal)
- Lunch: Paleo lunch pack. 1 banana (105 cal), 1 apple (95 cal), 1 chicken (239 cal), hazelnuts (628 cal), 2 boiled eggs (156 cal), 200 g green pepper (40 cal)
- Snack: Chips of baked courgette (49 cal), cut into a thin squash. Install slices on a paper towel and remove excess water. Let's sit for 20 minutes. The bowl is mixed with 5ml coconut oil salt (40 cal), pepper (40 cal) and courgette slices (52 cal). Place in an oiled pan and bake at 110 ° C for 2.5 hours or until it is crisp.
- Dinner: Spaghetti squash (31 cal)

Tuesday

- Breakfast: Egg Cake (115 cal). Combine 12 eggs (936 cal) with 450 g of peanut sausage and 2 small onions (56 cal), 1/2 green pepper (20 cal) and as many mushrooms (22 cal) as you want. Tilt in a container and bake for 30 minutes at 175 ° C. Cool the residue.
- Snack: Beef (250 cal)
- Lunch: Avocado (160 cal) salad with tomato (17.69 cal), and add baby spinach leaves (23.18 cal) and tomatoes.
- Snack: Apple (95 cal) and 1 tbsp almond butter (614 cal)
- Dinner: Tomato and artichoke chicken

Wednesday

- Breakfast: Almonds (576 cal) and berries (57 cal) with coconut milk (230 cal). (Tip: Buy frozen berries to save costs.)
- Snack: Large banana (89 cal) with 1 tbsp almond butter
- Lunch: Paleo super salad (152 cal). Tilt a large number of small spinach leaves with a small handful of walnuts (654 cal), 10-12 strawberries (48 cal) (sliced), two boiled eggs and soft vinegar (18 cal).
- Snack: Full of almonds (576 cal)
- Dinner: Chicken (239 cal), mushrooms (22 cal) and cauliflower puree (25 cal)

Thursday

- Breakfast: Pepper (40 cal)-baked eggs (90 cal) with turkey bacon (382 cal). Heat some coconut oil (862 cal) and bake two eggs inside the pepper rings. Serve with two slices of Turkish bacon.
- Snack: Carrot sticks (41.35 cal) with guacamole (155 cal)
- Lunch: Whitefish wraps (172 cal). Grilled white fish fillets (cod, Pollak, hake). Put it in the surrounding salad (152 cal), add ½ avocado (sliced) and rub with lime (30 cal) and coriander (23 cal).
- Snack: Smoked salmon (208 cal) on slices of cucumber (15.54 cal)
- Dinner: Tomato and artichoke chicken residues

Friday

- Breakfast: Scrambled eggs (148 cal)
- Snack: A small number of grapes (67 cal)
- Lunch: Hot Chicken (76 cal) and Courgette Salad (66 cal)
- Snack: Beef (250 cal)
- Dinner: Spaghetti squash (31 cal) left over

Saturday

- Breakfast: Catching Turkish sausage (400 cal). Peel 60g turkey sausage, 1 sweet potato (86 cal) and 90g brussel idiot into pieces. Pull it all 3 eggs (75 cal) until the sausages (301 cal) are all cooked.
- Snack: Banana (89 cal)

- Lunch: Chicken salad fajitas (48 cal)
- Snack: Full of almonds (576 cal)
- Dinner: Chicken (239 cal), mushrooms and cauliflower puree

Sunday

- Breakfast: Scrambled eggs (148 cal)
- Snack: Banana (89 cal), blueberries (57 cal), pineapple (50 cal) and cinnamon smoothies (247 cal). Mix half of the banana, a handful of frozen blueberries, half frozen pineapple, a handful of cabbage (25 cal), 1 tbsp of almond butter and 200 ml of water in a blender.
- Lunch: Tomato and artichoke chicken residue
- Snack: Cucumbers (15.54 cal)
- Dinner: Garlic (148.9 cal) and herb pork(100 cal) minced meat (332 cal) with dessert potato (190 cal).

In line with this, many diseases and pathologies of the modern era were almost non-existent in the Paleolithic. Men hunted, and women gathered the fruits of nature. Everything came from nature without cultivation or intensive farming. Today modern man is overweight and out of shape, while our ancestor was more muscular and had a lower percentage of body fat. Why not try a return to the origins? According to the paleo diet cereals - for example - are not well assimilated by our body, since we are not made to take them. Most contain - indeed - gluten and lectins, to which many people are intolerant. Less consumption of refined and industrial foods - promises a paleo diet - will lower diabetes, celiac disease, and high cholesterol!

Chapter Eleven
Salt and the Paleo Diet

Salt consumption, such as carbohydrates, protein and fat, is surrounded by controversy and conflicting opinions from the medical community. The medical community generally believes that salt intake leads to high blood pressure and increases the chances of getting heart disease.

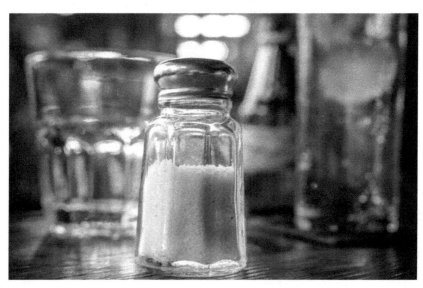

Indeed, there are a plethora of studies to suggest that this is true, especially for people who eat exclusively with industrial products. On the other hand, most research on salt consumption is done on refined and fluorinated salt, not natural, unprocessed sea salts.

The strict Paleo diet excludes salt but is it not a mistake for our health not to consume quality natural salt in the Paleo diet?

Salt is a compound of sodium and chloride. Both are electrolytes that regulate extracellular fluid volume and play a role in muscle and nerve function.

Let's look at the effects of a salt intake adapted especially during Paleo diets that promote natural foods and exclude the cooked dishes that are often too salty to enhance their taste.

The accumulation of scientific evidence shows that a low-salt diet can actually lead to severe health implications and higher overall mortality, especially in conditions such as heart disease and diabetes.

A study published in the New England Journal of Medicine with a population that consumed a moderate amount of sodium of between 3,000 and 6,000 mg/day was in better health than those who consumed either more or less than 3,000 to 6,000 mg/day. A conclusion that supports the beneficial effects of moderate sodium consumption on health.

Another study has shown that salt restriction is associated with insulin resistance, elevated triglycerides, and elevated stress hormones. Cardiac surgeon Richard Pooley does not restrict the salt or saturated fat consumption of his cardiac patients because he has not detected salt-related factors as causes of their problems.

- **Medical Dangers of Too Much Sodium**

Salt has a fascinating history; in the past, it was sometimes used as a currency or a reason to start a war. It is simply a natural component of seawater, left by evaporated water. Salt in the diet provides the body with the right sodium intake, which is essential for life. Although the excess of this can cause a serious imbalance in your body, increasing the risk for several potential serious medical problems.

- **Sodium / Salt**

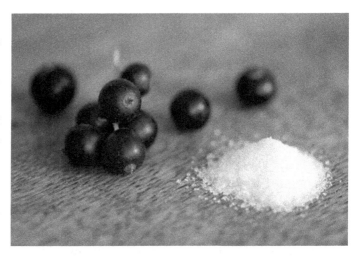

Chemically, table salt is sodium chloride, a crystalline compound that contains 40% sodium. Sodium is also a natural component found in many common foods. Our nerves use sodium to produce impulses and to contract muscles. Since sodium retains water, the body also uses it to regulate the amount of fluid in the blood, organs, and tissues. When the body contains too much sodium, the kidneys produce more urine to expel it. However, if you consume large amounts of sodium, your kidneys may not be able to handle all the excesses, risking to keep too much sodium in your body. This can cause several problems that increase the risk of serious diseases.

- **High Blood Pressure**

Blood pressure is an indicator of how much pressure the blood uses to radiate artery walls, heart rate and the times when the heart is "relaxed." The amount of blood in your circulation is called "blood volume," and is an important factor that determines blood pressure. When more salt is eaten than the kidneys can handle, excess salt retains water and increases the "blood volume," increasing blood pressure. High blood pressure can cause serious health problems, especially because it does not produce early symptoms.

- **Heart Disease and Stroke**

When too much sodium is consumed and the blood pressure is too high, over time, the extra pressure can make the vessels less elastic and more susceptible to the accumulation of fatty deposits called plaques. The health consequences of these include atherosclerosis or hardening of the arteries. In atherosclerosis, the vessels tighten, and their walls thicken, creating extra work for the heart and increasing the risk of heart attack, heart attack, and stroke. According to the Harvard School of Public Health, increased salt intake can cause a 23% increase in the aforementioned diseases and increase heart disease by 14%.

- **Other Issues**

According to Harvard experts, those who consume too much salt can have osteoporosis, or thinning of the bones, as salt abuse tends to wear down calcium from the bones. High sodium intake can also increase the risk of developing stomach cancer, according to the World Cancer Research Fund and the American Institute for Cancer Research.

- **Lowering Salt Intake**

The National Heart, Lung and Blood Institute recommends that healthy adults consume no more than 2,400 milligrams of sodium per day, equivalent to 6 grams of table salt or about 1 teaspoon. If you have or are at risk of high blood pressure, it is recommended to consume only 1,500 milligrams a day. Use less salt at the table or replace it with herbs and spices without salt, and check the seasoning labels for the amount of salt content. Choose fresh fruits and vegetables and rinse salads and canned vegetables before serving. Choose low-salt products and check the wording for "hidden" salt on product labels, avoiding sodium bicarbonate, sodium nitrate, sodium citrate, and sodium benzoate.

To consume salt in the Paleo diet in a reasonable way here are the 7 points to respect:

- Use natural and unrefined sea salt. Pollution of the seas and oceans around the world means that some salts may contain mercury and other toxic heavy metals.
- Always salted your food after tasting it to avoid adding too much salt.
- If you have a Paleo diet based on mostly raw organic products, quality meats with outdoor animals and seafood using quality salt this will enhance the taste and cover your body's salt needs.
- If you drink enough water, adding a pinch of quality sea salt to every liter of water you drink will help maintain electrolyte levels and optimal energy levels.
- If you generously salty your food or eat processed foods, your water needs to be reduced or not salted as this can actually cause more harm than good and have adverse effects on your health.
- Athletes who experience a significant loss of electrolyte through perspiration, with the use of quality sea salt on their food and in water avoid this deficit of electrolytes and maintain high energy levels.

Balance disorders, head turning (due to low blood pressure) is a symptom related to low level of electrolyte. This can often be avoided by following the guidelines below.

The Paleo diet is naturally diuretic by the high consumption of vegetables, and it is essential to have a supply of water and sufficient salt.

If you suffer from weakness, constipation, fatigue, cramps, headaches, head turning when you get up, add natural salt, without additives, non-fluorinated, unrefined to your water and your diet. You can also supplement electrolytes or drink bone broths to avoid these inconveniences.

In summary, ban refined salt from your diet and promote moderate consumption of natural sea salt or quality salt flower as part of a Paleo food style.

Chapter Twelve
Paleo Diet and Exercise

Paleo diet and exercise are reminiscent of an adventurous life. The sporting discipline consists in pushing back its physical and mental limits by homo sapiens fitness exercises coupled with a "natural" diet.

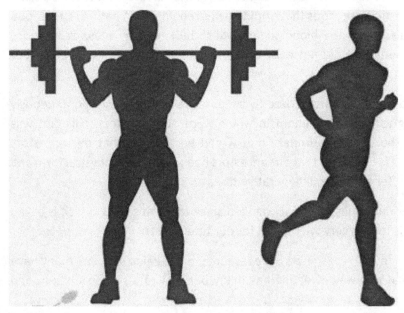

Machines, connected objects, and weights are dropped. The idea is to put the body in motion by producing natural gestures, ideally barefoot, like our ancestors who fled or hunted the buffalo: walk, run, jump, balance, crawl, climb, lift, carry, throw, catch, swim or defend yourself with the least possible effort. The exercises aim to give a slender and harmonious silhouette. Even if the wilderness is the privileged framework of training to explore all kinds of obstacles, the practice of paleo-fitness finds its place in gyms. Adepts learn how to walk quadruped for 100 meters, to lift weights and loads of different shapes, to run barefoot, to find balance, to jump obstacles, to climb trees.

Eating as in Paleolithic times excludes all grain and dairy products, but also all legumes, starchy vegetables such as potatoes, fatty meats, salt, sugar and of course all processed products and beverages soft. Like our hunter-gatherer ancestors, we adopt lean meats, poultry, fish, seafood, fruits and vegetables low in starch and all kinds of nuts and seeds (almond, sunflower, etc.). The paleo diet can lose up to 1 kilo of fat per week.

The Paleolithic diet, or Paleo, aims to revive the eating habits of the men of the Paleolithic, whose energy needs approach that of athletes: they too were extremely active and subjected to constant physical efforts. It is still possible to feed on all those foods that primitive men could find in nature. These food choices also allow the blood sugar level to be kept low, avoiding all those refined foods that did not exist in the Paleolithic but often appear on our tables.

Indeed, this diet is characterized by a diet made naturally and spontaneously according to the environment in which were our ancestors. This diet was revived. The most appropriate diet would be the diet that our ancestors adopted. It is described that our ancestors had an excellent physical form and did not suffer from any degenerative disease.

And since our genes have not changed since then, this food, which is called Paleolithic food is very well suited for our time.

Since then, many researchers have researched this Paleo diet, and many have shown that this way of eating has many benefits to a person's health and physique.

Moreover, the paleo diet has already been used as a remedy for certain diseases such as multiple sclerosis. A Paleolithic diet is a diet that does not necessarily mean eating meat or fish as we know.

After seeing the basics of Paleo nutrition and its health benefits, we will focus on the complementary activity that can be integrated into our daily life as a modern man. We will talk here about Paleo Fitness and the basic principles of this type of training.

The idea of these principles is to exercise daily to get closer to the life of our ancestors. This type of training does not require a gym membership or other accessories but just a little motivation.

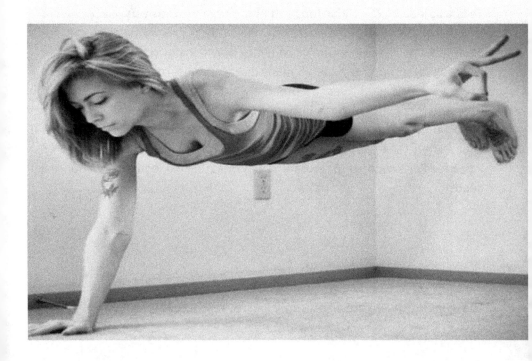

The basic idea of Paleolithic food is that our organism has very specific needs in terms of nutrition and that the way we eat in our modern societies is not at all suitable. Because of the discrepancy between our real needs and what we bring to our bodies via food, many diseases appeared when they did not exist in the Paleolithic men. To prove it, studies are looking into the case of hunter-gatherer tribes that still feed in traditional ways. The individuals who make up these groups are far less affected by these diseases. On the other hand, when they adopt our mode of feeding, their health suffers quickly. Paleo feeding proposes to return to a way of eating inadequacy with our real needs.

To summarize there are 4 basic principles to respect:

Principle 1: Move A Lot but at A Slow Pace

This seems simple enough in principle, but we can see that modern man does not work anymore. The means of transport allowed him to get rid of this activity to a point where, for some, it does not work anymore.

The idea is to gradually reintegrate the walk into your daily life. It's not complicated in principle, just put it. In the beginning, you have to go gradually by going on small distances (a few kilometers are enough per day).

Think of walking or hiking as something natural, without feeling the effort.

The march is advised, the Paleo man would never run, except when he was hunted.

Regarding the environment, it is obvious that a natural environment lends itself perfectly. Also, favor an environment that is not flat to increase the intensity of the activity.

Principle 2: Preventing Sport from Becoming an Obligation

The Paleo man did not need to go to the latest fashionable gyms to be "physically fit." This is all the modern man created who has deformed him, the food but also all the daily facilities that no longer make him practice any exercise. And when he is not satisfied with his situation and considers that he has to get back in shape, he begins to practice exercises on specialized machines.

Why not stop the problem at source? For that, it is enough to have a healthy diet (Paleo) and to practice daily exercises throughout the day. Do not hesitate to walk, carry, climb stairs, cycle and everything that fits in your day and you can practice.

Principle 3: Lift Heavy Objects

You'll understand if you are not a fan of gyms. You can consider using objects such as rocks, trees, tires, or dumbbells to practice the wearing of objects. You can even consider exercises that make you carry your weight (Pumps). This is the kind of exercise that simulates the body's natural movements.

If you do this kind of exercise regularly and you pair it with the Paleo diet you will maintain your muscle tone.

Principle 4: Accelerate The Pace, Once in A While

There are different ways to practice acceleration. The goal is to recreate the situation that the Paleo man knew when he was in danger and pushed him to go to the top of his performances.

If you are familiar with running, start with 100-400 meter sprints.

For cyclists, you can either find long flat areas and make an acceleration to practice maximum effort for 1-2 minutes.

For swimmers, you also have to swim at the height of your ability to feel the maximum effort.

The acceleration should be done once a week to be effective, but if you do not feel it as an effort, you can do it 3-5 times a week.

HEALTH BENEFITS

They are multiple and can be summarized as follows: the needs of the body are better covered; it works so better. In addition, it receives a lesser amount of substances that are harmful or useless, and it is only better. Paleolithic nutrition could, therefore, reduce the occurrence of many diseases among which we can find cancers, cardiovascular diseases, degenerative and autoimmune diseases, bone, joint problems, diabetes, etc. It would be possible to live in better health and probably longer.

THE BENEFITS FOR BODYBUILDING

Thanks to a diet rich in micro-nutrients, the body is less subject to deficiencies and can, therefore, be more efficient. This is reinforced by an intake of alkalizing foods that are supposed to help the body maintain an adequate acid-base balance for muscle growth. Consuming a greater amount of Omega 3 is also a valuable aid in building muscle.

These same parameters are beneficial to avoid losing too much muscle during a diet whose goal is the melting of body fat.

However, many critics focus on the difficulty of gaining weight in Paleolithic mode because the carbohydrate intake would be insufficient. But, the Paleolithic diet is not necessarily low in carbohydrates. The intake of fruits and vegetables, as well as tubers, can cover the caloric and carbohydrate needs of muscle building.

In addition, it is possible to pick some less problematic cereals such as buckwheat and basmati rice if the needs are too great. Nothing prevents you from making a correct weight gain.

Chapter Thirteen
How to make Trouble-Free Paleo Diet Recipes

In this chapter, you will be exposed to nice recipes that you can enjoy in recent days. These are everything you need to prepare very special bread, as it is a low carb, paleo, vegan and gluten-free recipe.

What do all these big words mean? Let's see it together.

What is Paleo Nutrition

As previously stated in other chapters; the term "paleo" derives from the Paleolithic, the prehistoric era prior to the advent of agriculture. According to supporters of the Paleo Diet, the only way to eat healthy according to the needs of our body is to feed ourselves following a "caveman diet."

A purist returns to the origins that consider only the foods that can be hunted and fished valid and genuine; foods that can be collected in nature. In the Paleo diet, cereals and sugars are not allowed, and therefore fewer carbohydrates are consumed automatically. Dairy products are also excluded, while sweet potatoes and sometimes rice can be eaten.

When we talk about "Low Carb," we refer to a real lifestyle that is based on the principle of consuming a few carbohydrates in one's diet. It is about eliminating as much as possible the consumption of sugar and high-carbohydrate foods (bread, pasta, rice, potatoes, corn).

The philosophy of this diet is based on the principle that, by eating few carbohydrates, you do not experience glycemic peaks: there is no increase in blood glucose, there is no greater release of insulin, and consequently hunger attacks are avoided sudden and frequent. Having consistently low insulin levels is a great help for both those suffering from diabetes and those trying to lose weight. As said earlier, however, this diet is a real lifestyle rather than a temporary "diet." You can talk about low carb feeding up to a maximum carbohydrate consumption of around 100-150g per day.

The low carb diet allows the following foods:

- Vegetable at will (preferably in season)
- Meat (preferably from grazing cattle)
- Fish and seafood
- Eggs (preferably organic)
- Quality oils and fats (coconut oil and extra virgin olive oil)
- Seeds and nuts
- Seed flour and nuts (almond flour, walnut flour, flax seed flour)
- Dairy product
- Fruit
- Alternative sweeteners of natural origin (xylitol, stevia)
- Legumes (to be consumed occasionally)

The foods to avoid are:

- Cereals
- Sugar and sweets
- Pasta, bread, pizza and baked goods prepared with cereal flours

- "Light" products, usually rich in sugar or synthetic sweeteners
- Rice and potatoes
- Sunflower oil, corn oil, margarine
- Sugary drinks
- alcohol

The paleo is dedicated to the promotion of low carbohydrate for low carb diets, therefore suitable for diabetics, sports people, people with weight problems or simply for those who choose a natural diet without cereals and sugar. This means that better nutrition leads us to a better life.

The principles are:

- Eat healthy for a healthy life
- Exclusion of refined and sweetened products
- Back to nature, back to the origins
- Consumption of healthy and natural products and naturally produced ingredients

The Recipe for Paleo Veg Low Carb and Gluten-Free Bread

In the beginning, you might be a bit skeptical about the taste and consistency of this bread. And instead, you had to change my mind completely!!! The taste is very good, especially if you are already used to eating whole meal bread rather than white flour.

The consistency of the crumb is soft, while the crust remains crispy and crumbly as soon as it comes out of the oven. This bread is also kept fresh and soft for several days.

To better appreciate freshly baked bread, you could also spread on it an 85% strawberry fruit compote and a hazelnut chocolate cream, both vegan, gluten-free and with no added sugar. Really delicious!

We hope you found this useful and interesting to discover new things about particular choices in terms of nutrition and health.

And also If you think that following the paleo diet means giving up on putting tasty and various foods on your plate, you will have to change your mind soon. In fact, within the Paleo world, we find a large quantity of food to cook in an often fanciful way, which with a little imagination and the right seasonings will turn into really inviting dishes. The Paleo diet is inspired by the way our ancestors feed themselves, by foods that have not undergone technological processes to become edible. This does not mean that it is unattractive or tasteless. Indeed, Paleo cuisine is based on the use of spices that are often rich in virtues for our body.

One of the spices most used in Paleo cuisine, besides turmeric, is chili. This special ingredient, rich in vitamins and mineral salts, has always been known for its beneficial effects on blood pressure and blood circulation. The recipes that use this remedy for the body range from first courses to meat, passing through fish and side dishes.

A first course characteristic of the Paleo diet includes a sauce based on fresh sliced tomatoes, onion and chili. As a base, you can use spaghetti made from zucchini passed through the blade with triangles smaller than the vegetables sliced. Put the onion and a little oil in a non-stick pan. As soon as the onion starts to fry, add the spaghetti with zucchini and the fresh tomato. Cook for a few minutes, add the chili and serve on the table. This recipe is particularly suitable on summer days when the external heat makes our body desire particularly fresh foods, rich in water and easily digestible.

On colder days, an exquisite onion soup will be particularly welcome. To make it, start by roughly cutting the onions and placing them inside a pot with high sides. Then add salt and a glass of water — Cook for a quarter of an hour in a covered pan. When the onions are soft, remove from the heat, add a tablespoon of coconut flour and pass the mixture into the blender. Add the oil and freshly ground chili pepper.

When autumn comes, why give up on serving a delicious soup that encompasses all the colors and scents of this season?

Made with yellow pumpkin and porcini mushrooms, you can make some cream rich in beta-carotene and minerals that will prove to be valuable antioxidants that can counteract free radicals. A small addition of chili will make pumpkin cream and porcini mushrooms a real natural medicine for blood circulation.

Among the meat-based main courses, you must try the breaded chicken morsels, made with chicken breast, lemon, almond flour, salt, chili pepper, and parsley. After reducing the chicken breast to small pieces, place it in a bowl and add the seasonings. Finally, dip in the almond flour for a light breading before laying the morsels in a non-stick pan. If you love spicy dishes, do not miss to try the jalapeno peppers stuffed with guacamole, ideal to serve as a snack for a break or a party. Do not miss even the deviled eggs, quick to prepare and cheap, which will be particularly appetizing if you add a pinch of pepper to the pan during cooking.

Hence, fish-based dishes are the ones that are best combined with chili. Anchovies, eels, squid, groupers, snappers, but also mollusks such as sea date, octopus, cuttlefish, and squid will be even more delicious if you add a pinch of chili pepper during cooking. In this way, you will make dish rich in B vitamins (in particular vitamin B12), iron, iodine, zinc, and selenium, contributing at the same time to the health of your arteries.

On the other hand, many people eat bread at every meal. The paleo diet is focused on fish, eggs, and vegetables. Bacon and red meat even find their place at breakfast. The paleo diet allows paleo bread, but the bread is unfortunately only a small component of paleo diet menus. That said, you do not have to go without bread. Provided of course that it is paleo bread.

It is often wrongly thought that paleo bread tastes more like cake than bread. By choosing the right recipes, you will see that the paleo bread can make a delicious bread. Here are additional 3 recipes of paleo bread to try.

Paleo Bread Recipe 1: Banana Bread

Rich in nutrients, this paleo bread is good for your health and easy to prepare. The banana gives it a sweet taste. When you have tasted it, this paleo bread will be part of your favorite recipes.

Ingredients - What is needed to make banana bread?

- 6 eggs (468 cal)
- 1 teaspoon of Celtic sea salt
- 2 ripe bananas (210 cal)
- 2 tablespoons of honey (128 cal)

- 1 teaspoon of vanilla extract (12 cal)
- 80 ml of coconut milk (187 cal)
- 130 g of coconut flour (120 cal)
- 90 g of almond flour (150 cal)
- 1 tablespoon baking soda
- 2 tablespoons raisins (299 cal)

Preparation

- Preheat the oven to 180 ° C.
- Grease the bread pan (size 28 cm).
- Beat the eggs and add a little salt.
- Crush the bananas and add them to the eggs.
- Add honey (304 cal), vanilla extract (288 cal), coconut milk, coconut flour, and almond flour.
- Add the bicarbonate and mix well.
- Stir in the raisins and bake for 45 to 55 minutes.

Paleo Bread Recipe 2: Avocado Bread

A surprising bread whose taste will make you forget other bread. You will never want to return to the bread you ate before starting the paleo diet.

Ingredients - What is needed to make avocado bread?

- 3 avocados peeled and cut into pieces (966 cal)
- 6 eggs (468 cal)
- 5 tablespoons of honey (75 ml) (320 cal)
- 4 tablespoons freshly squeezed orange juice (60 ml) (28 cal)
- 150 g of almond flour (150 cal)
- 75 g of coconut flour (120 cal)
- 1 tablespoon of baking powder (6 cal)
- 1 teaspoon of cinnamon (6 cal)
- 1 teaspoon of black pepper (7 cal)
- 1 teaspoon of Celtic sea salt

Preparation

- Preheat the oven to 180 ° C.
- Grease the bread pan.
- In a blender, mix avocados, eggs, honey, and orange juice.
- Add the baking powder, coconut flour and almond flour, salt, and herbs.
- Mix and pour the mass into the mold.
- Bake for about 20 to 25 minutes.

Paleo Bread Recipe 3: Dried Fruit Bread

Nuts are very good for health and give the bread a delicious taste. Recommended in almost all types of diet, nuts have become very popular in recent years. Naturally, it is necessary to opt for nuts that are raw and natural, that is to say, not grilled and without salt. You can even choose the nuts that you prefer.

Ingredients - What is needed to make dried fruit bread?

- 1 tablespoon of honey (64 cal)
- 5 eggs (390 cal)
- 150 g of almond flour (150 cal)
- 50 g of coconut flour (120 cal)
- 50 g of finely ground nuts (e.g., almonds (576 cal), walnuts (654 cal) or hazelnuts (628 cal).
- 1 teaspoon of Celtic sea salt
- As a garnish, you can opt for 200 g of figs, dates (282 cal) or other dried fruits

Preparation

- Preheat the oven to 170 ° C.
- Grease the bread pan.
- Beat the eggs well. Add the other ingredients and pour the mixture into the mold.

- Cover the mold with aluminum foil and bake. After 40 minutes, remove the aluminum foil and cook the paleo bread 40 minutes more.

Other options

The paleo diet requires work. No question of grabbing a sandwich quickly done well in the morning. Your daily diet will require a little energy. People with busy work weeks struggle to follow the paleo diet. When you have a family, the time you have in the morning is limited. One idea is to prepare your paleo bread at the weekend and put some to freeze, but there are other options. Many paleo breakfast recipes contain eggs, fish and fruits. But why not try it? That said, many people will soon feel the need for paleo bread.

Chapter Fourteen
How to Lose Weight and Avoid Obesity with the Paleo Diet +3 weeks Plan

If the Paleo diet interests you, here is all the information on How to Lose Weight and Avoid Obesity with the Paleo Diet +3 weeks Plan. After reading, you will know everything and the better approach about this famous diet and its effectiveness.

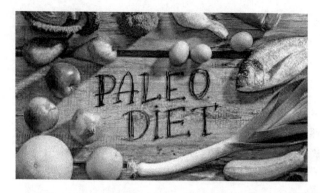

During the paleo diet, proteins, oleaginous and vegetable are to be preferred unlike dairy products, sweetened, processed and cereals that are to be avoided. The paleo diet upsets our eating habits. But by following it, you will be able to lose weight, avoid obesity and improve your overall health.

Moreover, according to the analysis of bones found by anthropologists and the study of populations living according to the prehistoric way of life, hunter-gatherers of the Paleolithic era were in better health. They were notably thinner, taller (for that time), muscular and did not suffer from osteoporosis.

But from the Neolithic period, the health of our ancestors has deteriorated with the arrival of agriculture. Over the past fifty years, obesity and diseases such as diabetes or cardiovascular diseases have developed considerably due to the appearance of industrial dishes.

According to the scientists who wrote about the Paleo diet, this diet would allow us to lose weight, be more energetic and prevent the onset of certain diseases.

The current diet is slightly different from that of our ancestors. The first difference concerns the number of calories per day: for the paleo diet, it is 3000 against 1800 (for a woman) and 2600 (for a man) today.

In terms of nutrients, the paleo diet is richer in protein: between 25 and 29% against 15 to 17% today. At the time, our ancestors consumed more protein, especially animal. But they also ate plants (between 600 and 1600 g / day).

In contrast, the Paleolithic diet is much lower in carbohydrates: between 39 and 40% against 49 and 59% currently. But why such a gap? The only source of sugar for our ancestors was fruits, berries or roots. They did not eat dairy products or cereals. As a result, they consumed fewer carbohydrates than today. In addition, the carbohydrates consumed in the past were of better quality (there were no refined sugars unlike today).

At the level of lipids, the levels are almost equivalent between the ancestral and modern food: between 30 and 39% for the first and between 33 and 37% for the second. If today we eat almost as much fat as our ancestors, the latter is however different: the ratio omega-3 / omega-6 was lower: 0.6 to 0.83 formerly against 11 today.

The 3 Weeks Plan Main Principles of This Ancestral Slimming Program

The Paleo diet is based on three main principles which are:

- Consume fruits and vegetables at will (they must be starch-free).
- Eat seafood and lean meats.
- Ban cereals, legumes, processed foods, and dairy products.

The Main Objectives of This 3 Weeks' Plan

In addition to helping you lose your extra pounds and bring you energy, the Paleo diet has other goals, such as:

- It helps to increase muscle mass in athletes.
- It improves the general state of health.
- It reduces the feeling of tiredness.
- It decreases digestive disorders and acid reflux.
- It prevents the appearance of certain diseases such as osteoporosis, cardiovascular diseases, type II diabetes, high blood pressure or hypertriglyceridemia.
- It relieves certain diseases such as rheumatoid arthritis.
- It decreases morning stiffness and clears the sinuses.

How Does This Diet Lead to Weight Loss?

First of all, be aware that the removal of processed products and starchy foods leads to weight loss. In addition, the proteins and fibers present in the paleo diet cause a sensation of satiety. This effect makes it possible to fill a desire to eat. Fibers have another advantage: they facilitate digestion and are beneficial for intestinal transit.

By following the paleo diet to the letter, you will be able to lose weight. But how long should it be followed? Ideally for life. However, the consistency of 3 weeks' plan will go a long way. Indeed, its positive actions are noted quickly (from its inception). This is why many people decide to follow this lifestyle in the long term.

How Not to Regain Weight in The Event of a Stoppage of the Diet?

If you decide to stop the paleo diet, you are not immune to weight gain. Indeed, by stopping, you will resume a "diet today" with the reintroduction of sweet products or industrial. To avoid taking back your lost pounds (or more), try to keep a diet high in lean protein.

The paleo diet does not only allow to lose weight. It is also beneficial for getting back into shape, preventing the onset of certain diseases and protecting one's health. Coupled with a sport (walking, weight lifting, sprinting ... as hunter-gatherers used to do), this ancestral diet can also increase muscle mass, reduce body fat and improve body composition.

Adopting the Paleo diet is also changing your diet and leaving out the current one. This involves the removal of sweets, hamburgers, chips, pizzas and other modern dishes. By setting up these new habits, you will be able to lose weight.

Also, the number of meals and the proportions are free. It is only recommended to eat when hunger is felt until you are full.

To keep up with the Paleo diet and to be effective, it is important to respect the main principles and rules. Among its rules, there are permitted and prohibited foods. To guide you and avoid a misstep, here's what you need to eat and banish from your diet.

Authorized foods

Seasonal vegetables

Vegetables should be consumed at all meals and in large quantities. Very satiating, they are ideal to quickly feel a sense of satiety. Tip to optimize micronutrients intake: consume vegetables of different colors.

Seasonal fruits

Foods allowed as part of the paleo diet you can eat it for dessert or as a snack. Among those to favor, there are raspberries, strawberries, berries, blueberries, and blackberries, because they are rich in anti-oxidants and little sweet.

Lean meats

Among the low-fat meats, you can find poultry, veal (escalope, for example) or pork tenderloin. By eating lean meat, you can stock up on protein!

The fish

As part of the Paleo diet, eat fish twice a week. Why? Because they are rich in omega-3 and therefore beneficial to protect the heart. They also have an interesting anti-inflammatory effect.

Eggs

Rich in protein, eggs are to be consumed between 3 and 5 times a week. And rest assured! Their cholesterol intake will have little impact on your blood cholesterol level.

Seeds and nuts

Almonds, nuts, hazelnuts, sunflower seeds ... Add them to your salads or take as a snack. Seeds and nuts provide the body with good unsaturated fats, fiber, protein, and other minerals and vitamins.

The oils

If our ancestors did not cook, incorporating olive, rapeseed and nut oil into your "paleo" diet is a good idea to season your dishes. In addition, these oils provide the body omega-3 or 9 beneficial for him and your health!

Pleasure foods

In the pleasure food category, the paleo diet allows for low-sugar dark chocolate with more than 70% cocoa and one to two glasses of wine a day.

The cereals

Rye, barley, corn, wheat, oats should not be included in your diet. According to experts in Paleolithic food, humans are not "genetically equipped" to feed on cereals. Rich in carbohydrates, cereals would lead to a sharp increase in blood glucose and therefore a significant production of insulin. However, an increase in this production is responsible for weight gain, or even the development of heart disease and diabetes.

Cereals should be avoided if you follow the paleo diet. But if you love them, do not exceed 80 - 120 grams per day.

Dairy products

In the Paleolithic era, dairy products did not exist. Yet our ancestors had strong bones. This was due to the calcium provided by fruits, vegetables, and vegetables. If you follow the paleo diet, your consumption of dairy products must be limited. But if you want to integrate, choose unsweetened and natures.

Sweet foods

Pastries, cookies, sweets are to be banned because they increase blood sugar levels and insulin production. In addition, they lack micronutrients.

Processed and industrial products

Already prepared dishes, industrial foods high in fat, salt and sugars are also banned from your diet. Of poor quality, they contain additives, dyes, and preservatives bad for health. Another negative point: they lead to weight gain.

Chapter Fifteen
3 weeks Diet Plan

Here Is The Perfect 3 Weeks Paleo Diet Plan:

Day 1

BREAKFAST: TOMATO SAUSAGES

Ingredients:

- 300 gr. of sausage
- 300 gr. of fine tomato pulp
- 3 tablespoons of extra virgin olive oil
- a quarter of white onion
- 2 tablespoons of chopped parsley
- 1 bay leaf
- Salt to taste
- black pepper to taste

Preparations:

1. Cut the sausage into small pieces but do not remove the skin.
2. Thinly slice the onion.
3. Put a pan on the heat, pour the extra virgin olive oil and add the onion, leaving it to dry for a few minutes.
4. Then add the sausage in pieces and let it flavor and color for a few minutes.
5. When the sausage has browned, often turn the pieces of sausage so that they are well seasoned.

6. Once the cooking sauce has thickened, add the fine tomato pulp, the chopped parsley and the bay leaf.
7. Season with salt and freshly ground pepper, mix well and continue cooking over medium heat with a covered pan for about ten minutes.
8. The sausage is ready to be served and served on the table with its cooking sauce. Enjoy your meal!

Nutritional Information:

Calories 746 Kcal | Fats 63 g | Carbohydrates 17 g | Protein 24 g

LUNCH: HAM AND MANGO

Ingredients:

- 100 g raw ham 9 slices
- 1 mango 300 g

Preparation:

- Before starting the ham must be cut into very thin slices, just like a sheet of paper, to better savor its taste. In addition, you can get more slices but pay the same price.
- Remove the peel of the mango, recover the pulp and remove the stone. Lay the mango and ham slices on the serving plate or directly on the individual plates.

Nutritional Information:

for 1 portion (150g): Calories: 140 | Grassi 2 g: 3% | Saturated 0.7 g | + Trans 0 g: 3% | Cholesterol 10 mg | Sodium 630 mg: 26% | Carbohydrates 18 g: 6% | fibers 2 g: 7% | Net carbohydrates 16 g | Protein 14 g | Vitamin A: 8% | C vitamin 4: 8% | Iron: 3%

DINNER: ASPARAGUS AND TOMATOES WITH VINAIGRETTE

Ingredients:

- 16 asparagus 320 g
- 1 tomatoes 120 g
- 2 tablespoons extra virgin olive oil 30 mL
- 1 tablespoon lemon 1/2 lemon
- 1/2 clove garlic
- 1 pinch 0.2 g

Preparation:

1. Prepare the asparagus and blanch them in a saucepan with salted water for about 10 minutes, depending on the size, for al dente cooking.
2. Remove the asparagus from the water with tongs or a slotted spoon (the asparagus tips are delicate and could break if they were drained directly into a colander). Pass the asparagus under cold water to stop cooking and fix the color. So let the asparagus spread over the individual plates for about ten minutes.
3. Prepare the tomatoes: cut them and place them on the plates next to the asparagus.
4. In a small bowl pour the oil and lemon juice. Salt and pepper. Beat this vinaigrette with a fork until it is emulsified. Squeeze the garlic and add it to the vinaigrette. Pour over the vegetables and serve.

Nutritional Information:

for 1 portion (190g): Calories 160 |Grassi 14 g 22% |Saturated 2 g |+ Trans 0 g 10% |Cholesterol 0 mg |Sodium 20 mg 1% |Carbohydrates 8 g 3% |fibers 3 g 12% |Net carbohydrates 5 g |Protein 3 g |Vitamin A 36% |C vitamin 33% |Iron 9%

SNACK:

Slice of 1 cup raw carrots, stir into 1 tablespoon tahini, and finish off the veggie mix with 1/2 tablespoon flaxseeds. Total calories: 89

Day 2

BREAKFAST: BEEF PARMENTIER WITH SWEET POTATO AND CORIANDER

Ingredients:

- Coriander 0.5 boot (10 g)
- Yam About 500 g (600 g)
- Potatoes About 200 g
- Rocket 0.5 tray (50 g)
- Ground beef 180 g
- Shallot 0.5 (15 g).

In your kitchen: Salt |Pepper |Olive oil |Vinegar of your choice |1 x Oven |1 x Baking dish |1 x Saucepan |1 x Sauteuse |1 x Colander

Preparation:

1. Take care of the potatoes. Preheat your oven to 240 ° C and boil a pot of salt water to cook the potatoes and sweet potato. Meanwhile: Peel the potatoes and sweet potato. Cut them into pieces (about 1cm). Immerse them in boiling water and cook 15/20 min until crushed.
2. Peel and chisel (small dice) the shallot. In a pan, heat a drizzle of olive oil over medium-high heat. Fry the shallot with the ground beef 7 min. Salt, pepper. Suggestion: add a pinch of cumin, cinnamon or chilli. Rinse and chop coriander (whole, stems are eaten). Rinse, drain the arugula and place it in a salad bowl in the fridge. In a bowl, prepare a vinaigrette with a drizzle of olive oil, vinegar, salt and pepper.
3. When the potatoes and sweet potato are cooked, drain them, put them back in the pan and mash them. Add Salt, pepper.
4. When the beef is cooked, add the coriander and arrange it in a gratin dish. Cover with mashed potatoes. Suggestion: sprinkle with breadcrumbs. Bake 10 min until it is hot.
5. As you sit down, season the salad with vinaigrette. Serve beef parmentier with sweet potato and hot coriander, accompanied by salad.

Nutritional Information:

Calories 627 kcal |13.5g Mast. fat |18g protein |0.2g Salt

LUNCH: SANDWICH ROLLED WITH TUNA AND AVOCADO

Ingredients:

- 8 small tortillas or 4 large
- 1/2 cucumber
- 2 ripe avocados
- 2 tuna cans
- 1 tomato
- 1 bunch of flat parsley
- 2 tablespoons olive oil
- 1 teaspoon strong mustard
- salt and pepper
- curly lettuce

Preparation:

1. Cut the avocados into 2 and using a spoon, remove all the flesh and pour into a large bowl. With the back of the spoon, crush the pieces as much as possible to form a paste.
2. Peel the cucumber and cut into small cubes before mixing with the avocado. Cut the tomato into quarters, then remove all the flesh and grains (they would bring too much liquid to the mixture). Cut the quarters into small slices and pour them into the bowl.
3. Chop the parsley and add to the mixture. Drain the tuna carefully, crumble it with a fork and add it to the mixture.
4. Pour the olive oil and the mustard, salt and pepper, then mix well the preparation so that it is homogeneous.
5. On a clean board, lay the first tortilla. Place a little of the mixture in the middle, about 4 tbsp. soup. Add a few lettuce leaves on top, then fold both sides. Then fold down the bottom edge and finish rolling all the tortilla.
6. Cut the roll in 2 and if necessary, fix it with a toothpick. Repeat the process until there are no more ingredients.

Nutritional Information:

Amount Per Serving: Calories 326.8 |Total Fat 12.4 g |Saturated Fat 1.4 g |Polyunsaturated Fat 1.4 g |Monounsaturated Fat 6.4 g |Cholesterol 35.0 mg

|Sodium 605.5 mg |Potassium 563.8 mg |Total Carbohydrate 11.0 g |Dietary Fiber 11.7 g |Protein 26.1 g |Calcium 7.6 %

DINNER: FRIED CAULIFLOWER RICE

Ingredients:

- 1 head cauliflower cut into 4 large pieces
- 1 cup chicken broth
- 2 tablespoons sesame oil
- 2 green onions sliced
- 1 clove garlic minced
- 1 teaspoon grated ginger
- 2 chicken breasts minced
- 1/2 cup frozen peas
- 1/2 cup diced carrots
- 1/2 teaspoon sea salt
- 1 egg beaten

Preparation:

1. Put the cauliflower pieces in your Instant Pot with the broth and close it. Set the timer to 10 minutes, and close the lid.
2. When it's done, remove the cauliflower pieces and set aside. Pour the broth out of the pot, and set it to the sauté setting. Add the sesame oil, green onions, ginger, and chicken.
3. Cook until the chicken is browned.
4. Add the cauliflower back to the pot and mash until it breaks up into rice sized pieces. Stir in the peas, carrots, egg, and salt, and put the lid back on. Turn off the pot, cover, and 5. let sit for 5 minutes.
5. Stir and serve.

Nutritional Information:

There are 95 calories in 1 cup of Cauliflower Fried Rice. Calorie breakdown: 46% fat, 31% carbs, 23% protein.

SNACK:

Mango Energy Bites: These sweet treats are 100 percent all-natural. You can thank dried mangoes and dates, as well as a bit of unsweetened, shredded coconut. Hemp seeds also give them a bit of a protein boost. Per One Ball: 80 calories

Day 3

BREAKFAST: SLOW COOKED MEATLOAF

Ingredients:

- 1 pound grass-fed ground beef
- 1 egg
- 1 onion finely chopped
- 2 cloves garlic minced
- 1/4 cup almond flour
- 1 tablespoon Italian seasoning
- 1 teaspoon sea salt
- 1 8- ounce can tomato sauce no sugar added

Preparation:

1. Combine the beef, egg, onion, garlic, almond flour, and seasonings in a bowl and mix well. Form into a loaf and add to your slow cooker.
2. Cover and cook on low for 4-6 hours.
3. Before serving, top with the tomato sauce and cook for an additional 10 minutes.

Nutritional Information:

336 Calories; 9 Calories from fat; 9g Total Fat (3 g Saturated Fat; 3 g Monounsaturated Fat;) 106 mg Cholesterol; 670 mg Sodium; 38 g Total Carbohydrate; 3.2 g Dietary Fiber; 26 g Protein; 3.9 mg Iron; 6 mg Niacin; 0.5 mg Vitamin B6; 2.2 mcg Vitamin B12; 5.9 mg Zinc; 21.8 mcg Selenium; 111.1 mg Choline.

LUNCH: ROASTED VEGETABLES

Ingredients:

- 2 potatoes 400 g

- 2 carrots 200 g
- 1 onions 200 g
- 1 turnips 170 g
- 2 wedges garlic
- 2 sprigs rosemary 10 g
- 2 tablespoons olive oil 30 mL
- 1 pinch 0.2 g

Preparations:

1. Preheat the oven to 190 ° C.
2. Prepare the vegetables: cut into pieces of the same size approximately 1.5 cm thick and lay in a single layer on a generously oiled plate. Cover the vegetables with plaque oil. 3. Add the rosemary in tufts and the poached garlic after having crushed it with the flat part of the knife blade. Salt.
3. Cook in the center of the oven for 35-40 minutes until the vegetables are softened and become golden. Turn them over twice during cooking.
4. To serve.

Nutritional Information:

for 1 portion (210g): Calories 160 |Grassi 5 g 8% |Saturated 0.8 g |+ Trans 0 g 4% |Cholesterol 0 mg |Sodium 60 mg 3% |Carbohydrates 28 g 9% |fibers 4 g 17% |Sugars 6 g |Net carbohydrates 24 g |Protein 3 g |Vitamin A 55% |C vitamin 35% |Iron 9%

DINNER: LAMB VEGGIE STEW

Ingredients:

- 2 tablespoons olive oil
- 1 Onion sliced
- 1 Carrot sliced
- 1 Zucchini sliced
- 1 Green pepper sliced
- 1 pound lamb cubed
- 4 cups Chicken broth

- fresh chopped parsley for serving

Preparation:

1. Heat the oil in a large soup pot. Add the vegetables and cook until softened. Add the lamb and cook until lamb is browned. Stir in the broth and bring to a boil.
2. Reduce heat and simmer until lamb is tender. Serve topped with the chopped parsley.

Nutritional Information:

Calories 521 |54% Total Fat 35g grams |55% Saturated Fat 11g grams |Trans Fat 0.3g grams |32% Cholesterol 97mg milligrams |52% Sodium 1242mg milligrams |28% Potassium 991mg milligrams |8% Total Carbohydrates 23g grams |14% Dietary Fiber 3.6g grams |Protein 28g grams |95% Vitamin A |23% Vitamin C |8% Calcium |23% Iron

SNACKS:

Best Homemade Oven Beef Jerky: This beef jerky doesn't contain any added sugar and consists of a delicious blend of spices, like oregano, garlic powder, chile powder, and paprika. It's nice and chewy and high in protein with a whopping 20 grams per serving. Per serving: 124 cal, 3 g fat (1 g sat), 2 g carbs, 0 g sugar, 750 mg sodium, 0 g fiber, 20 g protein.

Day 4

BREAKFAST: ROAST BEEF WITH VEGETABLES

Ingredients:

- 2 carrots 200 g
- 2 potatoes 400 g
- 1 fennel 360 g
- 6 segments garlic
- 60 mL olive oil
- 1 pinch 0.2 g
- 1 kg boneless beef belly

- 2 tablespoons Dijon mustard 30 g
- 1 Teaspoon honey 7 g
- 125 mL red wine [optional]
- 2 teaspoons antique mustard (with whole grains) 10 g

Preparation:

1. Before starting keep the serving dishes warm by placing them on the hob. Preheat the oven to 160 ° C.
2. Prepare the vegetables by cutting them into uniform pieces of about 1.5 cm. Leave the garlic in shirt.
3. Heat half of the oil in a large frying pan and add all the vegetables, exclusion made for the garlic, and sauté over moderate heat until they take on color, for about 8 minutes.
4. Salt and pepper, then, remove the vegetables from the pan and transfer them to a dish.
5. Pour the remaining oil into the same pan and brown the roast until the sides are completely browned, or for 8-10 minutes. Transfer the roast to a baking dish, brush it with Dijon mustard, add salt and pepper. Put away the pan without cleaning it in order to preserve the meat juices and prepare the sauce. Put the vegetables and garlic cloves around the meat.
6. Cook in the center of the oven for about 50 minutes if you have a roast of about 1 kg or until the thermometer inserted in the meat indicates 70 ° C (perfect cooking). Take the pan out of the oven, place the roast on a cutting board, cover with aluminum and let it sit for 10 minutes. Leave the vegetables in the oven off. Peel the garlic cloves, crush them, reduce to puree and set aside.
7. Heat the honey over high heat in the previously used pan. Deglaze with the wine (optional) and add the mustard grains and the garlic cloves in puree. Cook everything for 1-2 minutes, stirring.
8. Remove the aluminum and finely slice the roast by cutting in a transverse direction. Serve the meat slices with the vegetables and the sauce on the hot plates.

Nutritional Information:

for 1 portion (320g): Calories 470 |Grassi 20 g 30% |Saturated 5 g |+ Trans 0.3 g 26% |Cholesterol 100 mg |Sodium 280 mg 12% |Carbohydrates 28 g 9% |fibers 5 g 20% |Net carbohydrates 23 g |Protein 45 g |Vitamin A 55% |C vitamin 31% |Iron 40%

LUNCH: BAKED GRILLED VEGETABLES

Ingredients:

- 3 parsnip 280 g
- 3 carrots 300 g
- 1 celeriac 650 g
- 3 tablespoons olive oil 45 mL
- 1 tablespoon Origan 2 g
- 1 pinch 0.2 g

Preparation:

1. Preheat the oven to 190 ° C. Grease a plate or baking pan generously.
2. Peel the vegetables and cut them into pieces of the same size (about 2 cm on each side). Place them in the pan without overlapping them. Mix them to coat them well with oil.
3. Add the oregano and a little salt and pepper.
4. Bake and cook until the vegetables are golden brown (35-40 minutes). Mix them twice during cooking to obtain a uniform result.
5. To serve.

Nutritional Information:

Calories 130 |Grassi 5 g 8% |Saturated 0.7 g |+ Trans 0 g 4% |Cholesterol 0 mg |Sodium 120 mg 5% |Carbohydrates 20 g 7% |fibers 4 g 17% |Net carbohydrates 16 g |Protein 2 g |Vitamin A 55% |C vitamin 25% |Iron 8%

DINNER: STEAK, EGGS, AND BROCCOLI

Ingredients:

- 3 tablespoons clarified butter
- 8 ounces sirloin steak cubed
- 2 green onions sliced
- 1 clove garlic minced

- 2 cups broccoli florets
- 2 eggs
- Sea salt and fresh ground pepper to taste

Preparation:

1. In a heavy, nonstick skillet, heat the butter to medium high heat. Add the steak and cook until well browned. Remove from pan and set aside. Add the green onions and garlic and cook for about a minute. Add the broccoli and cook for about 3 minutes. Move the broccoli to one side and add the eggs to the other. Cook the eggs to your liking and remove from the pan.
2. Add the steak back to the pan with the broccoli and stir until heated through. Serve the steak and broccoli topped with an egg.

Nutritional Information:

Calories 464 | Total Fat 29.1g 45% | Total Carbohydrates 8g 3% | Dietary Fiber 2.8g 11% | Protein 43g 86%

SNACKS:

Perfect Deviled Eggs: Deviled eggs are a great paleo snack. Plus, this recipe offers 12 variations on the classic to bring in even more flavor options. Some toppings include smoked paprika, sriracha and lime, lemon and chive, curry, peppered bacon, and avocado. Per serving: 55 cal, 4.4 g fat (1 g sat), 0.4 g carbs, 0.3 g sugar, 151.8 mg sodium, 0.1 g fiber, 3.2 g protein.

Day 5

BREAKFAST: BREAKFAST SWEET POTATO HASH

Ingredients:

- 1 large onion, sliced
- 3 tbsp olive oil, divided
- 1/2 tbsp ghee
- 2 Italian sausages, diced
- 2 sweet potatoes
- 3 tbsp fresh rosemary
- Salt and freshly ground black pepper, to taste

- 3 eggs

Preparations:

1. Preheat the oven to 425 degrees F. Line a baking sweet with parchment paper. Heat one tablespoon of olive oil and the ghee in a skillet over medium heat. Add the ohions and sprinkle with salt. Cook on low heat for 30-40 minutes, until dark brown and caramelized.
2. Meanwhile, peel the sweet potatoes and chop into bite-size pieces. Place into a large bowl with the remaining two tablespoons of olive oil and rosemary.
3. In a separate skillet, cook the sausages until browned. Add the cooked onions and sausages to the bowl with the sweet potatoes and toss. Season with salt and pepper.
4. Spread out the sweet potato mixture evenly onto the prepared baking sheet. Roast for 30-35 minutes until the potatoes are soft and browned. Either refrigerate overnight at this point or proceed to the next step.
5. Place the sweet potato hash into a cast iron skillet and make three small wells to crack the eggs into. Crack eggs into the skillet and season lightly with salt and pepper. Bake for 15-18 minutes at 425 degrees F until the eggs are set.

Nutritional Information:

Calories 419 kcal |Potassium 478.1 mg |Vitamin A 527.9 µg |Vitamin C 5.8 mg |Folic Acid (B9) 35.5 µg |Sodium 496.8 mg

LUNCH: TUNA AVOCADO LETTUCE WRAPS

Ingredients:

- 1 can tuna
- ½ very ripe avocado
- 2 tbsp paleo mayo
- ¼ cup green olives

- 2 tbsp diced green chiles
- 1 scallion
- 2 large leaves of green leaf lettuce

Preparations:

1. Cut olives in half and dice scallion.
2. Mash the avocado until it's a creamy consistency, and then mix with paleo mayonnaise.
3. Add in the tuna, olives, scallion, and diced green chiles to the avocado-mayonnaise mixture.
4. Place one scoop of tuna salad into a large leaf of lettuce, wrap, and enjoy!

Nutritional Information:

Calories 282 kcal |Potassium 486 mg |Vitamin A 54.7 µg |Vitamin C 29.7 mg |Folic Acid (B9) 62.4 µg |Sodium 527.6 mg

DINNER: BUTTERFLIED ROASTED CHICKEN

Ingredients:

- 1 whole chicken, patted dry
- 3 tbsp. melted Paleo cooking fat
- 3 tbsp. fresh rosemary, finely chopped
- 2 onions, peeled and quartered
- 4 carrots, peeled and sliced
- 2 bell peppers, chopped
- 2 lemons, halved
- Sea salt and freshly ground black pepper to taste

Preparations:

1. Preheat your oven to 400 F.
2. Place the chicken, breast-side down, on a cutting board. Cut along both sides of the backbone from end to end with kitchen shears and remove the backbone. Flip the chicken breast-side up, and open it like a book. Press firmly on the breasts with your palm to flatten.
3. Save the backbone for some homemade stock.

4. In a small bowl, combine the cooking fat and 2 tbsp. of the rosemary.
5. Rub the chicken with 2/3 of the fat/rosemary mixture and season the chicken to taste with sea salt and ground pepper.
6. Line a large baking sheet with aluminum foil.
7. Place the chicken on the baking sheet and surround it with the vegetables and the lemons.
8. Pour the remaining fat/rosemary mixture over the vegetables and season to taste.
9. Place the baking sheet in the oven and cook for 1 hour or until a meat thermometer reads 165 F in the thickest part of the breast.
10. Remove chicken from oven, squeeze some lemon juice over it, and serve

Nutritional Information:

Calories 310 Kcal |26% fat| 0% carbs |74% protein|Potassium 710.5 mg |Vitamin A 5.9 µg |Vitamin C 71.2 mg |Folic Acid (B9) 92.7 µg |Sodium 772.1 mg

SNACKS:

Homemade Strawberry Fruit Leather: 4 cups strawberries, hulled and chopped, 2 tbsp honey.

- Preheat the oven to 170 degrees F or the lowest oven temperature setting. Line a baking sheet with a Silpat mat. Place strawberries in a medium saucepan and cook on low heat until soft. Add in the honey and stir to combine.
- Use an immersion blender to puree the strawberries in the saucepan, or transfer to a blender and puree until smooth. Pour the mixture onto the Silpat-lined baking sheet and spread evenly with a spatula. Bake for 6-7 hours, until it peels away from the parchment.
- Once cooled, peel the fruit leather off the mat and use a scissors to cut the fruit leather into strips. Roll up to serve, and store in an airtight container.

Nutritional Information:

Calories 40 kcal |Potassium 119 mg |Vitamin A 0.8 μg |Vitamin C 44.7 mg |Folic Acid (B9) 18.4 μg |Sodium 1 mg

Day 6

BREAKFAST: DILL & LEMON BAKED SALMON IN PARCHMENT

Ingredients:

- 2 6-oz. salmon fillets
- 2 zucchini, halved lengthwise and thinly sliced
- 1/4 red onion, thinly sliced
- 1 tsp fresh dill, chopped
- 2 slices lemon
- 1 tbsp fresh lemon juice
- Extra virgin olive oil, for drizzling
- Salt and freshly ground pepper

Preparations:

1. Preheat the oven to 350 degrees F. Prepare two large pieces of parchment paper by folding them in half to crease. Then open the papers and lay flat.
2. On one side of the crease, place half of the zucchini, red onion, dill, and one lemon slice. Drizzle with olive oil and sprinkle with salt and pepper. Place a salmon fillet on top and drizzle with the lemon juice. Season with salt and pepper. Repeat with the second piece of parchment paper and remaining ingredients.
3. Fold the parchment paper over the salmon to close, making a half-moon shape. Seal the open sides by folding small pleats in the paper. Place the parchment packets on a rimmed baking sheet and bake for 15-20 minutes until the salmon is opaque. Serve warm.

Nutritional Information:

Calories 469 kcal |Potassium 1260.9 mg |Vitamin A 22.5 μg |Vitamin C 76.8 mg |Folic Acid (B9) 103 μg |Sodium 1057.3 mg

LUNCH: SPICY RED LENTIL CURRY

Ingredients:

- 2 Tbsp coconut oil
- 3 cloves garlic, minced (3 cloves yield ~1 1/2 Tbsp)
- 1 tsp minced ginger
- 1/2 cup diced carrots
- 3 Tbsp red curry paste (ensure vegan friendly)
- 1 6-ounce can tomato paste
- 2 cups low-sodium vegetable broth
- 1 cup water
- 2/3 cup dry red lentils (thoroughly rinsed in cold water + drained)
- 1-2 Tbsp coconut sugar
- 1/2 tsp ground turmeric
- 1/3 cup light coconut milk (optional)

FOR SERVING [optional]

- Cooked brown rice
- Pita or naan (omit if gluten free // check for vegan friendliness)
- Pickled red onion
- Fresh chopped cilantro

Preparations:

1. Thoroughly rinse lentils in a fine mesh strainer and set aside. If serving with brown rice, cook at this time using this method from Saveur.
2. Heat a large rimmed skillet over medium heat. Once hot, add coconut oil, garlic, ginger, and carrots. Sauté for 2 minutes, stirring frequently.
3. Add curry paste and sauté for 2 minutes, stirring frequently
4. Add tomato paste, vegetable broth, water and stir to combine. Then add lentils, coconut sugar, turmeric, and stir.
5. Bring to a simmer over medium heat, then reduce heat slightly to low (or medium-low), and gently simmer for 20 minutes, or until lentils are tender. Stir frequently to incorporate flavors, and add more vegetable broth as needed if the mixture becomes too thick.

6. An optional (but recommended) step: stir in coconut milk for additional creaminess, and to balance the heat of the curry paste.
7. Taste and adjust seasonings as needed, adding more turmeric for depth of flavor, coconut sugar for sweetness/flavor balance, or a pinch of salt for saltiness.
8. To serve, divide brown rice (optional) and lentils between 2-3 serving bowls and garnish with cilantro, pickled onions, and pita or naan for dipping (optional).

Nutritional Information:

Calories: 402 |Fat: 16.4g |Saturated fat: 10.9g |Sodium: 1340mg |Carbohydrates: 48g |Fiber: 15.9g |Sugar: 13.2g |Protein: 17.5g

DINNER: SPINACH AND MUSHROOM SALAD

Ingredients:

- salad spinach 120 g
- 6 Champignon mushrooms 80 g
- 1 tablespoon lemon 1/2 lemon
- 1/2 oranges 90 g
- 1/2 teaspoon Dijon mustard 3 g
- 2 tablespoons extra virgin olive oil 30 mL
- 1 pinch 0.2 g

Preparations:

1. Prepare the spinach and place them in a large bowl.
2. Prepare the mushrooms: finely slice and place in a small bowl. Season with salt and pepper and add half the lemon juice.
3. Peel half of the oranges and squeeze them to extract the juice. Put the zest and the orange juice in a small bowl and add the remaining lemon juice, mustard and oil. Salt and pepper. Beat everything with a fork until the vinaigrette is well emulsified.
4. Pour the vinaigrette over the spinach.
5. Peel the remaining oranges, cut into small pieces and add them to the spinach. Add the mushrooms. Stir and serve.

Nutritional Information:

Calories 160 |Grassi 14 g 22% |Saturated 1.9 g |+ Trans 0 g 10% |Cholesterol 0 mg |Sodium 50 mg 2 % |Carbohydrates 8 g 3% |fibers 2 g 7% |Net carbohydrates 6 g |Protein 3 g |Vitamin A 86% |C vitamin 54% |Iron 11%

SNACKS:

Homemade Paleo Protein Bars: These protein bars are rich and filling, and they're also gluten-, grain-, and dairy-free. With egg white protein and almond butter as main ingredients, they provide almost 11 grams of protein per bar. Add some delicious chocolate chips to make them feel indulgent and sweet, without compromising on nutrition. Per serving: 221 cal, 10.4 g fat (2 g sat), 23.4 g carbs, 16.2 g sugar, 133.2 mg sodium, 3.9 g fiber, 10.7 g protein.

Day 7

BREAKFAST: BROCCOLI EGG BAKE

Ingredients:

- 10 eggs
- 1/2 large onion, diced
- 2 medium zucchini, diced
- 1 medium head of broccoli, chopped
- 1 tsp salt
- 1/2 tsp freshly ground black pepper
- 1 tbsp fresh parsley, chopped

Preparations:

1. Preheat the oven to 350 degrees F. In a small bowl, whisk the eggs, salt and pepper. Stir in the chopped vegetables.
2. Grease a ramekin with coconut oil spray. Pour egg mixture into the dish and bake for 25-30 minutes or until the eggs are set. Remove from heat and let sit for 5 minutes before serving. Top with chopped parsley to serve.

Nutritional Information:

Calories 300 kcal |Potassium 891.4 mg |Vitamin A 198.6 µg |Vitamin C 155.8 mg |Folic Acid (B9) 164.8 µg |Sodium 762.8 mg

LUNCH: MEATBALL SANDWICH WITH ZUCCHINI BREAD & COCONUT CURRY SAUCE

Ingredients:

Meatballs

- ½ onion
- ½ tomato
- 4 cloves of garlic
- 1 egg
- 2 tbsp coconut milk
- 2 tsp sea salt
- ½ tsp black pepper
- ½ tsp paprika
- 1 lb. of grass-fed ground beef.

Zucchini bread and coconut sauce

- 1 onion
- 1 tomato
- 3 cloves of garlic
- 250g can coconut milk
- 4 very large zucchinis or 8 small ones (one per sandwich)
- 1 tsp sea salt
- 1 tsp curry powder
- 1 lemon
- Parsley

Preparations:

1. Preheat your over to 350 degrees. Line two roasting trays with aluminum foil.
2. Dice your tomato, onion and garlic. Set aside.
3. For the meatballs, crack open your egg and mix in tomato, onion, garlic, salt, black pepper and coconut milk.

4. It's time to get intimate with your creation. Put your beef into a mixing bowl and using your hands knead in the egg mixture. Shape into lovely little meatballs and place on roasting tray and put tray into heated oven for 20 minutes.
5. While your meatballs form into edible creations take your washed zucchini and slice them in half. Then dig out about 1/3 of the zucchini meat on one half and ½ from the top half.
6. Dice up the zucchini meat and add onion, tomato, garlic, salt, curry powder and add the coconut cream only (the water on the bottom is not needed so use it tomorrow for a tasty addition to a Crockpot chicken soup).
7. Mix everything and pour into your waiting zucchini tunnels. Remove your meatballs from the oven and place your zucchini into the oven at the same temperature.
8. Cook your guys for 20 minutes uncovered and then cover them with a sheet of foil for another 10 minutes.
9. Chop up your parsley and lemon wedges for plating.
10. Remove zucchini from oven and sprinkle some lemon juice on top. Nestle the meatballs into the deeper zucchini half place your second zucchini half on top, slice in half and serve with some parsley and lemon on the side for a mini salad garnish.

Nutritional Information:

Calories 234 kcal |Potassium 788 mg |Vitamin A 38.1 µg |Vitamin C 38.8 mg |Folic Acid (B9) 58.6 µg |Sodium 733.8 mg

DINNER: SALMON WITH PINEAPPLE JUICE

Ingredients:

- smoked salmon 100 grams
- pineapple Juice 100 grams
- walnuts 100 grams
- 1/2 teaspoons toasted sesame oil
- 1/4 teaspoon crushed red pepper
- 2/4 cup water

Preparations:

1. In small sauce pan combine pineapple Juice, water, sesame oil, and red pepper. Cook and stir over medium heat until thickened and bubbly. Cook and stir 2 minutes more
2. Rinse broiler. Rinse salmon and pat dry. Broil 4 inches from heat for 10 to 12 minutes. Place salmon on serving plates and sprinkle with little red pepper. Enjoy!

Nutritional Information:

Calories 467 | 78 mg cholesterol | 352 mg sodium | 20g carbohydrate |29g protein

SNACKS:

Energy Bars; Ingredients: 1 cup almonds, 1 cup dried cranberries, 1 cup pitted dates, 1 tbsp unsweetened coconut flakes, 1/4 cup mini dark chocolate chips.

Preparations: Combine all of the ingredients in a blender or food processor. Pulse a few times to break everything up. Then blend continuously until the ingredients have broken down and start to clump together into a ball. Using a spatula to scrape down the sides, turn out the mixture onto a piece of wax paper or plastic wrap. Press into an even square and chill, wrapped, for at least an hour. Cut into desired size of bars, wrapping each bar in plastic wrap to store in the fridge.

Nutritional Information:

Calories 345 kcal |Potassium 474.9 mg |Vitamin A 2.6 µg |Vitamin C 0.1 mg |Folic Acid (B9) 17.1 µg |Sodium 2.3 mg

Day 8

BREAKFAST: BREAKFAST BURRITOS

Ingredients:

For the tortillas

- 2 eggs
- 2 egg whites
- 1/2 cup water
- 4 tsp ground flaxseed

- Pinch of salt

For the filling

- 1 avocado, diced
- 1/4 cup red bell pepper, finely diced
- 1/4 cup onion, finely diced
- 1/4 cup baked tilapia or other protein
- Handful of spinach leaves
- 1 tsp coconut oil

Preparations:

1. In a small bowl, whisk together the ingredients for the tortilla. Preheat the oven broiler.
2. Heat a 10-inch non-stick skillet over medium heat and coat well with coconut oil spray. Pour half of the tortilla mixture into the pan and swirl to evenly distribute. Using a metal spatula, loosen the edges of the tortilla from the pan. Cook a couple of minutes until golden brown on the bottom, and then carefully slide the spatula under the tortilla to loosen it from the bottom of the pan. Do not flip yet.
3. Place the pan under the broiler for 3-4 minutes until the tortilla gets a little bubbly. Remove the tortilla from the pan, setting on a piece of aluminum foil. Repeat with other half of tortilla mixture.
4. After the tortillas are done broiling, preheat the oven to 400 degrees F. In a separate small pan, heat the coconut oil over medium heat. Add the onions and peppers and sauté for 5-8 minutes, until soft. Add the spinach into the pan and wilt.
5. Place all of the fillings down the center of the tortillas and wrap tightly. Place into the oven for 5-8 minutes to set the shape of the tortilla. Enjoy!

Nutritional Information:

Calories 315 kcal |Potassium 746.2 mg |Vitamin A 113.9 µg |Vitamin C 35.9 mg |Folic Acid (B9) 124.9 µg |Sodium 276 mg

LUNCH: HEALTHY PALEO NACHOS

Ingredients:

- 2 medium tomatoes, diced and seeded
- 2 tbsp fresh cilantro, chopped
- 2 cups guacamole
- 1-2 tbsp lime juice
- 2 tbsp green onions, chopped
- For the sweet potato chips:
- 3 large sweet potatoes
- 3 tbsp melted coconut oil
- 1 tsp salt

For the meat:

- 1 medium yellow onion, finely diced
- 1 tbsp coconut oil
- 1 green chili, diced
- 1 lb. ground beef
- 2 cloves garlic, minced
- 1 tsp smoked paprika
- 1/2 tsp ground cumin
- 1 tbsp tomato paste
- 12 oz. canned diced tomatoes
- 1 tsp salt
- 1/2 tsp pepper

Preparations:

1. To make the sweet potato chips, preheat the oven to 375 degrees F. Peel the sweet potatoes and slice thinly, using either a mandolin or sharp knife. In a large bowl, toss them with coconut oil and salt. Place the chips in a single layer on a rimmed baking sheet covered with parchment paper. Bake in the oven for 10 minutes, then flip the chips over and bake for another 10 minutes. For the last ten minutes, watch the chips closely and pull off any chips that start to brown, until all of the chips are cooked.
2. While the potato chips are baking, start preparing the beef. Melt the coconut oil in a large skillet over medium heat. Add the onion and chili to the pan and sauté for 3-4 minutes until softened. Add the ground beef and cook for 4-5 minutes, stirring regularly. Add the

garlic, diced tomatoes, tomato paste, and remaining spices and stir well to combine. Bring the mixture to a simmer and then turn the heat down to medium-low. Cook, covered, for 20-25 minutes, stirring regularly.

3. Stir the chopped tomatoes, lime juice, and cilantro into the beef mixture. Adjust salt and pepper to taste. Remove from heat.

4. To assemble the nachos, form a large circle with the sweet potato chips on a platter. Add the beef mixture into the middle of the circle, and then top with guacamole and green onions.

Nutritional Information:

Calories 375 kcal |Potassium 794 mg |Vitamin A 628.1 µg |Vitamin C 37 mg |Folic Acid (B9) 33 µg |Sodium 700.9 mg

DINNER: CROCK POT BEEF STEW

Ingredients

- 1 pound beef round steak, cubed
- 2 teaspoons olive oil
- 2 medium red onions, finely chopped
- 1 cup diced celery
- 2 cups diced ripe tomatoes
- 1 cup diced sweet potato
- ½ cup diced red pepper
- ½ cup diced yellow pepper
- 1 cup diced carrot
- 4 cloves of garlic, chopped
- 1 tbsp red wine vinegar
- 3 cups homemade beef stock or water
- 2 bay leaves
- 1 teaspoon minced fresh thyme
- 1 tablespoon minced fresh parsley
- salt and black pepper, to taste

Preparations:

1. In a large pan heat 2 tbsp olive oil over medium heat. Add the onion and garlic and saute for 2 minutes. Add beef cubes and cook until browned, about 3-4 minutes.
2. In a 6-qt slow cooker or French oven, combine meat and onion mixture, tomatoes, sweet potatoes, carrot, peppers, celery, bay leaves and stock. Cover with lid and cook on low
3. heat for 4 hours. Then uncover, stir in fresh herbs, season with salt and black pepper and serve.

Nutritional Information:

Calories 320 kcal |Potassium 1239.5 mg |Vitamin A 308.4 µg |Vitamin C 78.4 mg |Folic Acid (B9) 65.3 µg |Sodium 502.9 mg

SNACKS:

Paleo Antioxidant Berry Shake; Ingredients: 1/2 cup coconut milk, 1/4 cup cold water, 1/2 frozen banana, 1/2 cup frozen raspberries, 1/2 cup frozen blueberries, 1 tbsp chia seeds. Preparation: In a large cup (if using an immersion blender) or a blender, combine ingredients and blend until smooth. Add more water if necessary to reach desired consistency. Serve immediately.

Nutritional Information:

Calories 411 kcal |Potassium 667.2 mg |Vitamin A 5.4 µg |Vitamin C 31.9 mg |Folic Acid (B9) 46.5 µg |Sodium 21 mg

Day 9

BREAKFAST: BREAKFAST PIZZA

Ingredients:

For the crust

- 3 eggs
- 1 cup full-fat canned coconut milk
- 1/2 cup of coconut flour
- 2 tsp of garlic powder
- 1 tsp onion powder

- 1 tsp Italian seasoning
- 1/2 tsp baking soda

For the breakfast pizza

- 3 strips bacon
- 1/4 cup scallions, chopped
- 1-2 tomatoes, sliced thin
- 2 cups spinach
- 4 eggs
- 1 tbsp fresh parsley, chopped

Preparations:

1. Preheat the oven to 375 degrees F. To form the pizza dough, lightly beat the eggs and coconut milk in a bowl. Add in the coconut flour, baking soda, and seasonings and mix into a smooth batter.
2. Spread the batter onto a baking sheet lined with parchment paper, using a spatula to smooth into either a circle or rectangle. Bake for 18-20 minutes or until the top is golden brown. Remove from oven. Carefully flip over.
3. While the crust is baking, cook the bacon in a skillet over medium heat. Reserving the bacon fat in the pan, set the bacon aside to cool and crumble into pieces. Barely wilt the spinach in the leftover bacon fat.
4. Add toppings to the baked crust. Start with bacon, tomato, spinach, and scallions. Carefully crack eggs onto the crust. Sprinkle with parsley. Bake for 12-15 minutes more, just until the egg whites have set. Slice and serve warm.

Nutritional Information:

Calories 311 kcal |Potassium 366.8 mg |Vitamin A 168.3 µg |Vitamin C 8.5 mg |Folic Acid (B9) 66.5 µg |Sodium 368.4 mg

LUNCH: LOADED CAULIFLOWER BAKE

Ingredients:

- 1 medium cauliflower, cut into florets
- 2 cloves garlic minced
- 1 ½ tbsp olive oil
- 1 cup almond milk
- 1 ½ tbsp arrowroot flour
- 1/3 cup paleo approved store-bought or homemade mayonnaise
- 4 bacon slices, cooked and crumbled
- 1 tbsp chopped parsley
- salt, black pepper to taste

Preparations:

1. Preheat oven to 350°F.
2. Blanch cauliflower in a large pot of boiling water for 2 minutes.
3. Drain well and set aside.
4. To make the sauce in a skillet heat the olive oil over medium heat.
5. Add garlic and cook for 30 seconds.
6. Add the arrowroot flour and stir until golden.
7. Add the milk and bring to a low simmer, stirring until combined.
8. Stir in the mayonnaise and season with salt and pepper.
9. Add drained cauliflower and toss to combine.
10. Transfer the mixture into a casserole dish.
11. Bake for 30 minutes.
12. Remove from the oven, sprinkle with bacon and parsley and serve.

Nutritional Information:

Calories 354 kcal |Potassium 546.9 mg |Vitamin A 7.1 µg |Vitamin C 72.6 mg |Folic Acid (B9) 87.9 µg |Sodium 615.7 mg

DINNER: BEEF AND BROCCOLI STIR FRY

Ingredients:

- 1.5 lbs. sirloin, thinly sliced
- 4 tbsp coconut aminos, divided
- 4 tbsp red wine vinegar, divided
- 3 tbsp chicken broth

- 4 cloves garlic, minced
- 1 tsp arrowroot flour
- 1 tsp honey
- 1 tbsp ginger, minced
- 1/2 tsp sesame oil
- 1 head broccoli, cut into florets
- 4 carrots, diagonally sliced
- 3 tbsp coconut oil, divided

Preparations:

1. Place the sirloin in a small bowl with one tablespoon each of red wine vinegar and coconut aminos and toss to coat. Let marinate for 15 minutes at room temperature.
2. Meanwhile, whisk together 3 tablespoons each red wine vinegar, coconut aminos, and chicken broth. Stir in the garlic, ginger, arrowroot, honey, and sesame oil. Prepare a separate small bowl with 1 tablespoon of water and set it next to the stove along with the garlic sauce.
3. Melt 2 tablespoons of coconut oil in a large skillet over medium heat. Place the steak in the skillet in a single layer. The meat should sizzle; otherwise the pan is not hot enough.
4. Cook for 1-2 minutes per side to brown, and then transfer to a bowl.
5. Add the remaining tablespoon of coconut oil to the skillet. Stir in the broccoli and carrots, cooking for 2 minutes. Add the water to the skillet and cover with a lid. Let cook for 2-3 minutes, then remove the lid and cook until all of the water has evaporated.
6. Add the garlic mixture to the vegetables and stir to coat. Add the beef back into the pan and toss until the sauce thickens and everything is well coated. Serve immediately.

Nutritional Information:

Calories 379 kcal | Potassium 825.3 mg | Vitamin A 371.1 µg | Vitamin C 93.5 mg | Folic Acid (B9) 84.6 µg | Sodium 311.4 mg

SNACKS:

Homemade Baked Cinnamon Apple Chips; Ingredients: 1-2 apples (I used Honeycrisp), 1 tsp cinnamon.

Preparations: Preheat oven to 200 degrees. Using a sharp knife or mandolin, slice apples thinly. Discard seeds. Prepare a baking sheet with parchment paper and arrange apple slices on it without overlapping. Sprinkle cinnamon over apples. Bake for approximately 1 hour, then flip. Continue baking for 1-2 hours, flipping occasionally, until the apple slices are no longer moist. Store in airtight container.

Nutritional Information:

Calories 49 kcal |Potassium 101.1 mg |Vitamin A 2.9 µg |Vitamin C 4.2 mg |Folic Acid (B9) 2.8 µg |Sodium 1 mg

Day 10

BREAKFAST: GRANOLA

Ingredients:

- 1 cup cashews
- 3/4 cup almonds
- 1/4 cup pumpkin seeds, shelled
- 1/4 cup sunflower seeds, shelled
- 1/2 cup unsweetened coconut flakes
- 1/4 cup coconut oil
- 1/4 cup honey
- 1 tsp vanilla
- 1 cup dried cranberries
- 1 tsp salt

Preparations:

1. Preheat oven to 300 degrees F. Line a baking sheet with parchment paper. Place the cashews, almonds, coconut flakes and pumpkin seeds into a blender and pulse to break the mixture into smaller pieces.

2. In a large microwave-safe bowl, melt the coconut oil, vanilla, and honey together for 40-50 seconds. Add in the mixture from the blender and the sunflower seeds, and stir to coat.
3. Spread the mixture out onto the baking sheet and cook for 20-25 minutes, stirring once, until the mixture is lightly browned. Remove from heat. Stir in the dried cranberries and salt.
4. Press the granola mixture together to form a flat, even surface. Cool for about 15 minutes, and then break into chunks. Store in an airtight container or resealable bag.

Nutritional Information:

Calories 380 kcal |Potassium 296.9 mg |Vitamin A 0.1 µg |Vitamin C 0.4 mg |Folic Acid (B9) 16.6 µg |Sodium 173.9 mg

LUNCH: SHRIMP FRIED RICE

Ingredients:

- 1 tbsp coconut oil
- 1 cup white onion, finely chopped
- 2 cloves garlic, minced
- 8 oz. shrimp, peeled and deveined
- 1 medium carrot, chopped
- 1/2 cup peas
- 1/4 cup red bell pepper, finely chopped
- 2 cups cooked cauliflower rice
- 2 eggs, beaten
- Salt and pepper, to taste

Preparations:

1. Heat a wok or large pan over medium-high heat. Melt the coconut oil and add the onion and garlic to the pan. Cook for 3-4 minutes until the onion starts to soften. Add the shrimp and cook for 1 minute.
2. Add the carrot, peas, and bell pepper to the pan. Cook for 3-4 minutes, and then stir in the cauliflower rice. Clear a circle in the center of the pan and pour in the beaten eggs. Stir to scramble the

eggs and then combine with the other ingredients. Season with salt and pepper to taste.

Nutritional Information:

Calories 495 kcal |Potassium 365.2 mg |Vitamin A 214.1 µg |Vitamin C 23.5 mg |Folic Acid (B9) 56.4 µg |Sodium 614.1 mg

DINNER: SAUSAGE AND KALE PASTA CASSEROLE

Ingredients:

- 1 lb. Italian sausage
- 1 medium spaghetti squash, halved and seeded
- Extra virgin olive oil, for drizzling
- 1 large bunch of kale, de-stemmed, and chopped
- 1/2 red onion, sliced thin
- 1/3 cup chicken broth
- 1/2 cup coconut milk
- 1 clove garlic, minced
- 2 tsp Italian seasoning
- Salt and freshly ground pepper, to taste

Preparations:

1. Preheat the oven to 400 degrees F. Place the squash in the microwave for 3-4 minutes to soften. Using a sharp knife, cut the squash in half lengthwise. Scoop out the seeds and discard. Place the halves, with the cut side up, on a rimmed baking sheet. Drizzle with olive oil and sprinkle with salt and pepper. Roast in the oven for 45-50 minutes, until you can poke the squash easily with a fork. Let it cool until you can handle it safely. Then scrape the insides with a fork to shred the squash into strands.
2. Meanwhile, melt the coconut oil in a large oven-safe skillet over medium heat. Add the sausage and brown. Once cooked through, remove to a plate. In the same skillet, add the onion and sauté for 3-4 minutes. Next add the garlic, Italian seasoning, and kale and cook for 2-3 minutes to slightly wilt the kale. Pour in the chicken broth and

coconut milk and simmer for an additional 2-3 minutes. Remove from heat.

3. Stir in the cooked sausage. Add the spaghetti squash into the skillet and stir well to combine. Bake for 15-18 minutes, until the top has slightly browned. Serve hot.

Nutritional Information:

Calories 283 kcal | Potassium 409.7 mg | Vitamin A 160.8 µg | Vitamin C 40.6 mg | Folic Acid (B9) 58.9 µg | Sodium 451.6 mg

SNACKS:

Pumpkin Pie Smoothie; Ingredients: 1 frozen banana, 2 tbsp pumpkin puree, ½ cup unsweetened almond milk, ½ tsp vanilla extract, 1 tsp honey, 1 tbsp hemp hearts, ¼ tsp cinnamon, ¼ tsp cloves, ¼ tsp nutmeg.

Preparations: Combine all ingredients in a blender and process until smooth. I find it's easier on the blender if I break the frozen banana into smaller chunks before processing. Pour into a tall glass and enjoy with your favorite book, your favorite music, or both!

Nutritional Information:

Calories 244 kcal | Potassium 703.4 mg | Vitamin A 241.9 µg | Vitamin C 11.6 mg | Folic Acid (B9) 32.4 µg | Sodium 91.8 mg

Day 11

BREAKFAST: PUMPKIN PANCAKES

Ingredients:

- 1/4 cup pumpkin puree
- 3 tbsp almond milk
- 1 tbsp honey
- 3 eggs
- 1 tbsp coconut oil, melted, plus additional for pan
- 1 tsp vanilla
- 1/4 cup coconut flour
- 1 tsp cinnamon

- Pinch of nutmeg
- 1/2 tsp salt
- 1/4 tsp baking soda

Preparations:

1. In a large bowl, whisk together the dry ingredients – the coconut flour, cinnamon, nutmeg, salt, and baking soda. Then in a separate bowl, whisk together the wet ingredients – the pumpkin puree, almond milk, honey, eggs, oil, and vanilla. Add the dry ingredients to the wet ingredients. Stir together until just combined.
2. Heat a griddle or non-stick skillet to medium heat. Coat pan with coconut oil. Pour about 1/4 cup of batter onto the skillet. Cook for 2-4 minutes until the bottom is cooked through, and then flip. Cook for another 2-4 minutes until lightly browned. Repeat with remaining batter. Serve warm and enjoy!

Nutritional Information:

Calories 267 kcal |Potassium 181.6 mg |Vitamin A 341.7 µg |Vitamin C 1.4 mg |Folic Acid (B9) 35.3 µg |Sodium 355.8 mg

LUNCH: TACO SALAD WITH CREAMY AVOCADO DRESSING

Ingredients:

For the salad

- 2-3 cups shredded romaine lettuce
- 1/4 cup red onion, diced
- 3 tbsp sliced black olives
- 3 green onions, chopped
- 8 oz. ground beef
- 1 tsp chili powder
- 1/2 tsp ground cumin
- 1/4 tsp garlic powder
- 1/8 tsp dried oregano
- 1/8 tsp paprika
- Salt and pepper, to taste

For the dressing

- 1/2 avocado, pit removed
- 2 tbsp olive oil
- 1 tbsp lime juice
- 1 clove garlic, minced
- 1 tsp fresh cilantro, chopped
- 1 tbsp water
- Pinch of salt

Preparations:

1. 1.To make the dressing, blend the ingredients with an immersion blender or in a regular blender and process until smooth. Add more water if necessary to reach desired consistency, and taste for seasoning. Set aside.
2. Cook ground beef with seasonings over medium heat. Assemble salad by combining all of the salad ingredients in a large bowl. Toss well to combine. Top with dressing to serve.

Nutritional Information:

Calories 361 kcal |Potassium 574.6 mg |Vitamin A 202.7 µg |Vitamin C 10.8 mg |Folic Acid (B9) 99.2 µg |Sodium 482.9 mg

DINNER: ROASTED BUTTERNUT SQUASH SOUP

Ingredients:

- 1 large butternut squash (about 5 lbs)
- 1 green apple, sliced and cored
- 1 small yellow onion, chopped
- 2 carrots, chopped
- 3 tbsp olive oil
- 2 tsp cinnamon
- 1 1/2 tsp salt
- 1/2 tsp cumin
- 1 tsp chili powder
- 2 tbsp ghee
- 3 cups chicken broth

Preparations:

1. Preheat oven to 400 degrees F. In a large bowl, combine the butternut squash, olive oil, 1 tsp cinnamon, 1/2 tsp salt, and 1/2 tsp cumin. Mix together, coating the squash well.
2. 2.Spread out on a rimmed baking sheet.
3. Next, in the same bowl that the butternut squash was in, toss the apple slices, onion, and carrots to coat with the remnants. Place on a second rimmed baking sheet and add both baking sheets to the oven. Roast for 35-40 minutes until soft, stirring once.
4. Heat up ghee over medium heat in a large pot on the stove. Add the roasted ingredients and then the chicken broth. Add 1 teaspoon each of salt, cinnamon and chili powder.
5. Bring to a boil, then reduce heat to low and simmer, covered, for 20 minutes.
6. Using an immersion blender, combine the ingredients until smooth, or transfer to a blender to puree. Serve warm.

Nutritional Information:

Calories 380 kcal | Potassium 1652.1 mg | Vitamin A 2285.2 µg | Vitamin C 82.8 mg | Folic Acid (B9) 117.6 µg | Sodium 952.8 mg

SNACKS:

Energy Bars; If you made up the first batch of energy bars earlier in the week, you should still have a stash of them. Ingredients: 1 cup almonds, 1 cup dried cranberries, 1 cup pitted dates, 1 tbsp unsweetened coconut flakes, 1/4 cup mini dark chocolate chips.

Preparations: Combine all of the ingredients in a blender or food processor. Pulse a few times to break everything up. Then blend continuously until the ingredients have broken down and start to clump together into a ball. Using a spatula to scrape down the sides, turn out the mixture onto a piece of wax paper or plastic wrap. Press into an even square and chill, wrapped, for at least an hour. Cut into desired size of bars, wrapping each bar in plastic wrap to store in the fridge.

Nutritional Information: Calories 345 kcal |Potassium 474.9 mg |Vitamin A 2.6 µg |Vitamin C 0.1 mg |Folic Acid (B9) 17.1 µg |Sodium 2.3 mg

Day 12

BREAKFAST: KALE AND RED PEPPER FRITTATA

Ingredients:

- 1 tbsp coconut oil
- 1/2 cup chopped red pepper
- 1/3 cup chopped onion
- 3 slices crispy bacon, chopped
- 2 cups chopped kale, de-stemmed and rinsed
- 8 large eggs
- 1/2 cup almond or coconut milk
- Salt and pepper to taste

Preparations:

1. Preheat oven to 350 degrees. In a medium bowl, whisk the eggs and milk together. Add salt and pepper. Set aside.
2. In a non-stick skillet, heat about a tablespoon of coconut oil over medium heat. Add onion and red pepper and sauté for 3 minutes, until onion is translucent. Add kale and cook until it wilts, about 5 minutes.
3. Add eggs to the pan mixture, along with the bacon. Cook for about 4 minutes until the bottom and edges of the frittata start to set.
4. Put frittata in the oven and cook for 10-15 minutes until the frittata is cooked all the way through. Slice and serve.

Nutritional Information:

Calories 172 kcal |Potassium 236.9 mg |Vitamin A 179.6 µg |Vitamin C 32.6 mg |Folic Acid (B9) 54.7 µg |Sodium 254.4 mg

LUNCH: SHRIMP SCAMPI WITH ZUCCHINI PASTA

Ingredients

- 1 pound shrimp, peeled and deveined

- 3 garlic cloves , minced
- 1 ½ tbsp lemon juice
- ¼ tsp lemon zest
- 4 tbsp fresh parsley plus extra for garnish
- 1 small red serrano chili pepper, minced
- 4 tbsp olive oil
- 3 large zucchini
- ¼ tsp salt
- 1/8 tsp black pepper or to taste

Preparations:

1. Wash the zucchinis and slice them with a julienne slicer to get long noodles. In a small bowl combine the garlic, chili, parsley, lemon zest, salt, pepper and 1 tbsp of olive oil. Pour
2. about half of the parsley mixture over the shrimp and gently toss to coat. Marinate for 10 minutes.
3. In a large skillet, heat 2 tbsp of olive oil over medium heat. Add the shrimp along with the marinade and lemon juice to the skillet. Cook the shrimp for 3-4 minutes or until they
4. have turned pink. Remove the shrimp from the skillet. In the same skillet add the remaining olive oil, remaining parsley mixture and zucchini pasta and toss to combine. Cook for
5. about one or two minutes, then add in the shrimp and toss to combine. Season to taste.
6. Divide between serving plates and garnish with chopped parsley. Serve warm.

Nutritional Information:

Calories 492 kcal | Potassium 1559.8 mg | Vitamin A 172.1 µg | Vitamin C 93.6 mg | Folic Acid (B9) 162.2 µg | Sodium 1614.8 mg

DINNER: PALEO SLOW COOKER POT ROAST

Ingredients:

- 3 lbs. boneless beef roast, trimmed of fat
- 1 tbsp coconut oil
- 1 cup beef stock
- 5 carrots, peeled and diced
- 2 stalks celery, diced
- 1/2 large onion, sliced
- 3 garlic cloves, chopped
- 1 tbsp fresh parsley, chopped

For the spice rub:

- 1 tbsp freshly ground black pepper
- 1 tbsp ground coriander
- 2 tsp cinnamon
- 1 1/2 tsp salt
- 1/2 tsp ground clove
- 1/2 tsp ground allspice

Preparations:

1. Mix together the ingredients for the spice rub and massage into the roast. Heat the coconut oil in a large skillet over medium-high heat. Add the roast to the pan and let sear for 5 minutes. Flip and repeat with the other side. Transfer the roast to the slow cooker.
2. Add the carrots, onion, garlic, and celery to the slow cooker. Pour in the broth. Turn the heat on to low and cook for 6-7 hours, until the meat is tender. Serve hot sprinkled with chopped parsley.

Nutritional Information:

Calories 384 kcal |Potassium 791.8 mg |Vitamin A 322.9 µg |Vitamin C 4.4 mg |Folic Acid (B9) 33 µg |Sodium 612.3 mg

SNACKS:

Kale Chips; Ingredients: 1 bunch of kale, washed and dried, 2 tbsp organic olive oil, organic sea salt to taste.

Preparations: Preheat oven to 300 degrees. Remove the center stems and either tear or cut up the leaves. Toss the kale and olive oil together in a large bowl; sprinkle with salt. Spread on a baking sheet (or two, depending on the amount of kale). Bake at 300 degrees for 15 minutes or until crisp.

Nutritional Information:

Calories 28 kcal | Potassium 82.3 mg | Vitamin A 83.8 µg | Vitamin C 20.1 mg | Folic Acid (B9) 23.6 µg | Sodium 44.2 mg

Day 13

BREAKFAST: FRENCH TOAST WITH BLUEBERRY SYRUP

Ingredients:

- 1 loaf Paleo bread
- 1/2 cup almond milk
- 2 eggs
- 1/2 tbsp vanilla
- 1 tsp cinnamon
- 2-3 tbsp maple syrup

Preparations:

1. In a large bowl, whisk together the coconut milk, eggs, vanilla and cinnamon.
2. Heat a griddle or non-stick skillet to medium-high. Coat pan with coconut oil. Dip a slice of bread into the batter mixture to coat both sides, letting any excess drip off. Place the bread onto the pan and cook each side until slightly browned. Repeat with remaining bread. Serve warm.

Nutritional Information:

Calories 149 kcal | Potassium 112.5 mg | Vitamin A 17.3 µg | Vitamin C 0.1 mg | Folic Acid (B9) 53.2 µg | Sodium 269.9 mg

LUNCH: SPICY PEPPER CHICKEN STIR FRY

Ingredients:

- 2 lbs. boneless skinless chicken breasts, cut into 1-inch slices
- 2 tbsp coconut oil
- 1 tsp cumin seeds
- 1/2 each green, red, and orange bell pepper, thinly sliced
- 1 tsp garam masala
- 2 tsp freshly ground pepper
- Salt, to taste
- Scallions, for garnish

For the marinade

- 1/2 cup coconut cream
- 1 clove garlic, minced
- 1 tsp ginger, minced
- 1 tbsp freshly ground pepper
- 2 tsp salt
- 1/4 tsp turmeric

Preparations:

- 1.Place all of the marinade ingredients into a Ziploc bag. Add the chicken, close the bag, and shake to coat. Marinate in the refrigerator for at least 30 minutes, or up to 6 hours.
- 2.In a wok or large sauté pan, melt the coconut oil over medium-high heat. Add the cumin seeds and cook for 2-3 minutes. Add the marinated chicken and let cook for 5 minutes. Stir the chicken until it begins to brown, and then add the peppers, garam masala, and freshly ground pepper. Sprinkle with salt. Cook for 4-5 minutes, stirring regularly, or until the bell pepper is cooked to desired doneness. Serve hot.

Nutritional Information:

Calories 448 kcal | Potassium 952 mg | Vitamin A 40.6 μg | Vitamin C 20.3 mg | Folic Acid (B9) 35 μg | Sodium 660.6 mg

DINNER: PALEO STUFFED YELLOW SQUASH

Ingredients:

- 2 medium yellow squash
- 1 lb. ground beef
- 4 Roma tomatoes, diced
- 1 tsp coconut oil
- 1/2 large yellow onion, diced
- 3 cloves garlic, minced
- 1/2 tsp smoked paprika
- 1/2 tsp cumin
- 1/2 tsp ground coriander
- 1 tbsp tomato paste
- 1 tsp salt
- 1/2 tsp pepper
- 2 tbsp fresh parsley, chopped
- Extra virgin olive oil, for drizzling

Preparations:

1. Preheat the oven to 375 degrees F. Cut the squash in half lengthwise and use a spoon to scrape out the seeds. Place on a rimmed baking sheet with the cut-side up. Set aside.
2. 2.Melt the coconut oil in a large skillet over medium heat. Add the onion to the pan and sauté for 3-4 minutes. Stir in the garlic and cook for an additional minute. Add the beef to the pan and cook until no longer pink, stirring regularly.
3. 3.Add the diced tomatoes, along with the paprika, cumin, coriander, tomato paste, salt, and pepper. Stir well to combine.
4. 4.Spoon the beef mixture into the squash boats and lightly drizzle with olive oil. Bake for 25-30 minutes until the squash is tender. Serve warm, sprinkled with fresh parsley.

Nutritional Information:

Calories 464 kcal |Potassium 1307.5 mg |Vitamin A 87.8 µg |Vitamin C 37.8 mg |Folic Acid (B9) 61.1 µg |Sodium 700.5 mg

SNACKS:

Baked Paleo Chicken Tenders with Honey Mustard Dip: This healthier version of the crave-worthy crispy dish makes for a great paleo snack. By using almond flour, coconut flour, and almond milk for the batter—these protein-packed strips are way healthier than the original. But they're still packed with flavor thanks to a tasty array of spices and the honey mustard sauce that pairs perfectly. Per serving: 312 cal, 15.1 g fat, 9 g carbs, 0.9 g sugar, 4.6 g fiber, 33.6 g protein.

Day 14

BREAKFAST: PALEO STUFFED BREAKFAST PEPPERS

Ingredients:

- 2 bell peppers – your choice of color
- 4 eggs
- 1 cup white mushrooms
- 1 cup broccoli
- ¼ tsp cayenne pepper
- Salt and pepper, to taste

Preparations:

1. Preheat oven to 375 degrees Fahrenheit.
2. Dice up your vegetables of choice.
3. In a medium sized bowl, mix eggs, salt, pepper, cayenne pepper, and vegetables.
4. Cut peppers into equal halves. A tip: Try to buy peppers that are symmetrical and have somewhat flat sides – this makes it easier for them to balance while baking.
5. Core the peppers so that they're clean enough to add the filling.
6. Pour a quarter of the egg / vegetable mix into each pepper halve, adding more vegetables to the top to fill in any empty space.
7. Place on baking sheet and cook approximately 35 minutes or until eggs are cooked to your liking.
8. Serve and enjoy! I personally like mine with a dash of hot sauce on top.

Nutritional Information:

Calories 186 kcal |Potassium 640.9 mg |Vitamin A 343.5 µg |Vitamin C 193.5 mg |Folic Acid (B9) 130.2 µg |Sodium 666.5 mg

LUNCH: SHEET PAN CHICKEN THIGHS WITH SWEET POTATO AND BROCCOLI

Ingredients:

- 4 bone in chicken thighs
- ½ lemon, juiced
- 1 large sweet potato, peeled and cubed
- 1 medium broccoli head, cut into florets
- 3 tbsp olive oil
- 4 garlic cloves, minced
- 1 tbsp honey
- 1 tsp Dijon mustard
- ½ tsp salt
- ¼ tsp chili flakes
- black pepper to taste

Preparations:

1. Preheat oven to 425ºF.
2. In a bowl combine 1 tbsp olive oil, half of minced garlic, honey, Dijon mustard, _ tsp salt and chili flakes.
3. Add the chicken thighs and toss to coat.
4. Transfer the thighs into a baking tray and drizzle with marinade.
5. In the same bowl place the sweet potato, broccoli, remaining minced garlic, 2 tablespoons of olive oil and _ teaspoon salt. Season with black pepper to taste.
6. Toss to combine.
7. Arrange the veggies around the chicken in a single layer.
8. Bake for 30 - 40 minutes, turning halfway through cooking.
9. Drizzle the veggies with lemon juice and serve.

Nutritional Information:

Calories 532 kcal |Potassium 963.4 mg |Vitamin A 370 µg |Vitamin C 141.7 mg |Folic Acid (B9) 106 µg |Sodium 499 mg

DINNER: PALEO SHEPHERD'S PIE

Ingredients:

For the top layer

- 1 large head cauliflower, cut into florets
- 2 tbsp ghee, melted
- 1 tsp spicy Paleo mustard
- Salt and freshly ground black pepper, to taste
- Fresh parsley, to garnish

For the bottom layer

- 1 tbsp coconut oil
- 1/2 large onion, diced
- 3 carrots, diced
- 2 celery stalks, diced
- 1 lb. lean ground beef
- 2 tbsp tomato paste
- 1 cup chicken broth
- 1 tsp dry mustard
- 1/4 tsp cinnamon
- 1/8 tsp ground clove
- Salt and freshly ground black pepper, to taste

Preparations:

1. Place a couple inches of water in a large pot. Once the water is boiling, place steamer insert and then cauliflower florets into the pot and cover. Steam for 12-14 minutes, until tender. Drain and return cauliflower to the pot.
2. Add the ghee, mustard, salt, and pepper to the cauliflower. Using an immersion blender or food processor, combine the ingredients until smooth. Set aside.
3. Meanwhile, heat the coconut oil in a large skillet over medium heat. Add the onion, celery, and carrots and sauté for 5 minutes. Add in the ground beef and cook until browned.
4. Stir the tomato paste, chicken broth, and remaining spices into the meat mixture. Season to taste with salt and pepper. Simmer until

most of the liquid has evaporated, about 8 minutes, stirring occasionally.

5. Distribute the meat mixture evenly among four ramekins and spread the pureed cauliflower on top. Use a fork to create texture in the cauliflower and drizzle with olive oil.
6. Place under the broiler for 5-7 minutes until the top turns golden. Sprinkle with fresh parsley and serve.

Nutritional Information:

Calories 406 kcal | Potassium 1408.1 mg | Vitamin A 452.3 µg | Vitamin C 107.9 mg | Folic Acid (B9) 151.4 µg | Sodium 1140.9 mg

SNACKS:

Snickerdoodle Protein Balls: These snickerdoodle protein balls contain almond flour, cashews, and almond butter for a boost of protein. They also contain plenty of healthy fats thanks to those nutty ingredients—perfect for a mid-day snack. This recipe is ready in 10 minutes, and you can make a big batch at once to have for snacks throughout the week. Per serving (2 bite): 180 cal, 8 g fat (1 g sat), 21 g carbs, 18 g sugar, 120 mg sodium, 3 g fiber, 7 g protein.

Day 15

BREAKFAST: CHIPOTLE CHICKEN LETTUCE WRAPS

Ingredients:

- 2 tbsp extra virgin olive oil
- 1 lb. boneless skinless chicken breast
- 3 chipotle peppers
- Juice of 1 lime
- 4 tbsp adobo sauce
- 1/3 cup cilantro, chopped
- 1/2 red bell pepper, diced
- 2 scallions, thinly sliced
- 1 head lettuce, rinsed
- Salt and freshly ground pepper

Preparations:

1. Heat the olive oil in a large pan over medium heat. Sprinkle the chicken with salt and pepper on both sides and place in the pan. Cook for 5-6 minutes per side until the chicken is cooked through. Set aside and rest for 5 minutes, then shred.
2. In a food processor or blender, combine the chipotle peppers, adobo, cilantro, and lime juice. Blend until smooth.
3. Add the bell pepper, adobo mixture, and chicken to the sauté pan on low heat. Stir well to combine and cook for 3-4 minutes. Add the scallions to the pan. Spoon the mixture into lettuce wraps and serve.

Nutritional Information:

Calories 252 kcal | Potassium 647.5 mg | Vitamin A 433.2 µg | Vitamin C 59.5 mg | Folic Acid (B9) 58 µg | Sodium 878 mg

LUNCH: ROASTED PALEO CITRUS AND HERB CHICKEN

Ingredients:

- 12 total pieces bone-in chicken thighs and legs
- 1 medium onion, thinly sliced
- 1 tbsp dried rosemary
- 1 tsp dried thyme
- 1 lemon, sliced thin
- 1 orange, sliced thin

For the marinade:

- 5 tbsp extra virgin olive oil
- 6 cloves garlic, minced
- 1 tbsp honey
- Juice of 1 lemon
- Juice of 1 orange
- 1 tbsp Italian seasoning
- 1 tsp onion powder
- Dash of red pepper flakes
- Salt and freshly ground pepper, to taste

Preparations:

1. Whisk together all of the marinade ingredients in a small bowl. Place the chicken in a baking dish (or a large Ziploc bag) and pour the marinade over it. Marinate for 3 hours to overnight.
2. Preheat the oven to 400 degrees F. Place the chicken in a baking dish and arrange with the onion, orange, and lemon slices. Sprinkle with thyme, rosemary, salt and pepper. Cover with aluminum foil and bake for 30 minutes. Remove the foil, baste the chicken, and bake for another 30 minutes uncovered, until the chicken is cooked through.

Nutritional Information:

Calories 262 kcal |Potassium 246.4 mg |Vitamin A 23.3 µg |Vitamin C 14.1 mg |Folic Acid (B9) 12 µg |Sodium 297.4 mg

DINNER: BAKED SALMON WITH LEMON AND THYME

Ingredients:

- 32 oz piece of salmon
- 1 lemon, sliced thin
- 1 tbsp capers
- Salt and freshly ground pepper
- 1 tbsp fresh thyme
- Olive oil, for drizzling

Preparations:

1. Line a rimmed baking sheet with parchment paper and place salmon, skin side down, on the prepared baking sheet. Generously season salmon with salt and pepper. Arrange capers on the salmon, and top with sliced lemon and thyme.
2. Place baking sheet in a cold oven, then turn heat to 400 degrees F. Bake for 25 minutes. Serve immediately.

Nutritional Information:

Calories 507 kcal |Potassium 855.2 mg |Vitamin A 4.9 µg |Vitamin C 15.8 mg |Folic Acid (B9) 61.2 µg |Sodium 562.8 mg

SNACKS:

Sweet Potato Chips; Ingredients: 2 large sweet potatoes, 2 tbsp melted coconut oil, 2 tsp dried rosemary, 1 tsp pure sea salt. Preparations: Preheat oven to 375 degrees F. Peel sweet potatoes and slice thinly, using either a mandolin or sharp knife. In a large bowl, toss sweet potatoes with coconut oil, rosemary, and salt. Place sweet potato chips in a single layer on a rimmed baking sheet covered with parchment paper. Bake in the oven for 10 minutes, then flip the chips over and bake for another 10 minutes. For the last ten minutes, watch the chips closely and pull off any chips that start to brown, until all of the chips are cooked.

Nutritional Information:

Calories 29 kcal |Potassium 62.1 mg |Vitamin A 128.2 µg |Vitamin C 0.5 mg |Folic Acid (B9) 2.4 µg |Sodium 45.8 mg

Day 16

BREAKFAST: PALEO EGGS BENEDICT ON ARTICHOKE HEARTS

Ingredients:

Eggs Benedict:

- 4 eggs
- 1 egg white (use from Hollandaise Sauce Recipe below)
- 250 grams of bacon
- 4 Artichoke Hearts
- 3/4 cup of balsamic vinegar
- salt and pepper to taste

Hollandaise Sauce:

- 4 egg yolks
- 1 tbsp of lemon juice
- pinch of salt and paprika
- ¾ cup of melted ghee

Preparations:

138

1. Line a baking sheet with foil and set aside. Preheat your oven to 375 degrees. Deconstruct your artichokes and remove the artichoke hearts. Place the hearts in balsamic vinegar for 20 minutes.
2. For your Hollandaise Sauce, place a pot of water to simmer on your stove. Melt the ghee in a saucepan. Separate your eggs and place the yolks in a stainless steel cooking bowl. Hold on to the egg whites for the next step.
3. Remove your hearts from the marinade and place on cookie sheet, brush the tops of them with the egg white and then place your bacon over the artichokes as a second layer. Stick your tray in the oven for 20 minutes.
4. Back to the sauce, whisk the yolks with the lemon juice and then place your bowl over the simmering water. Slowly add in the ghee and bit of salt and continue to whisk until your sauce doubles in size and is silky. Set aside.
5. To poach your eggs, turn up the heat on your stove and let the same water get to a rolling boil. Crack your eggs one at a time into a ladle and the slide the egg into the water. Give them about a minute and a half and remove.
6. Now you are ready to assemble. Grab your artichoke hearts and bacon, then lay your poached egg and pour the Hollandaise silk on top.

Nutritional Information:

Calories 771 kcal |Potassium 437.8 mg |Vitamin A 451.4 µg |Vitamin C 6.4 mg |Folic Acid (B9) 70.2 µg |Sodium 602.6 mg

LUNCH: AVOCADO AND ENDIVE SALAD

Ingredients:

- 2 avocado 340 g
- 2 tablespoons chives [optional] 6 g
- 60 mL capers 40 g

- 4 spring onions
- 60 mL lime 2 files
- 2 tablespoons coriander [optional] 4 g
- 1 Belgian endive 150 g
- 2 tomatoes 240 g
- 1 pinch 0.2 g

Preparations:

1. Cut each avocado in half, remove the stone, remove the pulp with a spoon, transfer it to a bowl and crush it. Chop the capers, chives (optional) and spring onions. Add them to the bowl, crush well and mix together. Add the lime juice, salt and pepper to taste.
2. Distribute this purée in the center of the individual dishes and arrange the endive leaves all around alternating with the sliced tomato.
3. Garnish with chopped coriander leaves and serve immediately.

Kindly note: If the avocado puree is not served within an hour of preparation, carefully cover it with plastic wrap to prevent oxidation and refrigerate.

Nutritional Information:

for 1 portion (190g): Calories 130 |Grassi 9 g 15% |Saturated 1.4 g |+ Trans 0 g 7% |Cholesterol 0 mg |Sodium 310 mg 13% |Carbohydrates 12 g 4% |fibers 7 g 27% |Net carbohydrates 5 g |Protein 3 g |Vitamin A 22% |C vitamin 37% |Iron 7%

DINNER: BALSAMIC CHICKEN WITH ROASTED TOMATOES

Ingredients:

- 2 chicken thighs, bone-in
- 1 cup mushrooms, chopped
- 1/2 medium onion, chopped
- 1-2 tbsp extra virgin olive oil
- 3 tbsp balsamic vinegar
- Salt and pepper, to taste
- 1 pint cherry tomatoes
- 1 tbsp honey

- Fresh parsley, for garnish

Preparations:

1. Preheat the oven to 400 degrees F. Place the tomatoes on a baking sheet and drizzle with olive oil and honey. Sprinkle with salt and pepper and toss to coat evenly. Bake for 15-20 minutes until soft.
2. While the tomatoes are roasting, heat one tablespoon of olive oil in a large pan over low heat. Add the onions and mushrooms and cook for 10-12 minutes to soften and caramelize, stirring regularly. Clear a space for the chicken.
3. Season the chicken with salt and pepper and then place it in the pan. Add the balsamic, reduce the heat to low, and cover. Simmer for 15 minutes or until the chicken is cooked through. Every 5 minutes or so, spoon the sauce in the pan over the chicken.
4. To assemble, divide the tomatoes between two plates. Place one chicken thigh on each and then spoon the onions, mushrooms, and pan drippings over the chicken. Garnish with parsley.

Nutritional Information:

Calories 525 kcal |Potassium 920 mg |Vitamin A 108.1 µg |Vitamin C 26.8 mg |Folic Acid (B9) 42.3 µg |Sodium 1005.6 mg

SNACKS:

Almond Flour Pancakes: Pancakes make for a fun and tasty a.m. meal, and they're also perfect for a grab-and-go snack. The best part of these protein-packed, paleo pancakes— there are only five (yes, five) ingredients. Just mix almond flour, eggs, baking powder, coconut milk, plus vanilla, and you're good to go. Jazz them up with your fave toppings or mix-ins, like blueberries or walnuts. Per serving: 334 cal, 27.9 g fat (3.9 g sat), 11.2 g carbs, 2 g sugar, 5 g fiber, 14.4.5 g protein.

Day 17

BREAKFAST: ZUCCHINI AND CHORIZO PALEO BREAKFAST CASSEROLE

Ingredients:

- 3 large zucchini

- 1/2 red onion, chopped
- 1/2 cup mushrooms (optional)
- 5 eggs
- 2 links chorizo, casings removed
- 1 tsp salt
- Freshly ground black pepper, to taste

Preparations:

1. Preheat oven to 375 degrees F. Cook the chorizo in an oven-safe skillet over medium heat. Set aside.
2. Grate all of the zucchini and put into a large bowl. Using a paper towel, press some of the moisture out of the zucchini. In a separate bowl, beat the eggs with salt and pepper.
3. Combine all of the ingredients, including cooked chorizo, in the large bowl and mix together. You want to have enough eggs to coat the whole mixture. Warm about a 1/2 tablespoon of olive oil in the skillet over medium heat. Add the zucchini mixture into the pan. Cover and cook about 5 minutes until the eggs start to set on the bottom. Transfer to the oven and bake for 12-15 minutes, until the eggs are firm. Remove and let rest for 5-10 minutes, then serve.

Nutritional Information:

Calories 263 kcal |Potassium 862.4 mg |Vitamin A 110.5 µg |Vitamin C 44.5 mg |Folic Acid (B9) 87.2 µg |Sodium 796.8 mg

LUNCH: SLOW COOKED MUSHROOMS

Ingredients:

- 2 cups sliced mushrooms
- 2 sprigs thyme
- 2 cloves garlic smashed
- 1/4 cup olive oil
- 1/2 cup chicken broth
- 1/2 teaspoon sea salt

Preparations:

Put all ingredients in a slow cooker and cook over low heat for 2 hours. Serve immediately, or cool and store in the refrigerator until ready to serve.

Nutritional Information:

Calories: 410.5 |Sodium: 976.1 mg |Dietary Fiber: 1.7 g |Total Fat: 23.9 g

DINNER: COCONUT FLOUR CREPES

Ingredients

For the crepes

- 2 tbsp arrowroot flour
- 2 tbsp coconut flour
- ¼ tsp baking powder
- pinch of salt
- 1 egg
- 7 tbsp unsweetened almond milk
- olive oil for greasing

For the homemade sausage

- 1 pound lean ground pork or turkey
- ½ tsp salt
- ½ tsp black pepper
- ½ tsp dried thyme
- ½ tsp dried sage
- 1 tsp maple syrup
- ½ tsp onion powder
- ½ tsp cayenne pepper
- ¼ tsp red pepper flakes (optional)
- 2 tbsp olive oil

The rest of ingredients

- 1/3 cup tomato, chopped
- 4 fried eggs
- salt, black pepper to taste

Preparation:

1. To make the homemade sausage, heat the olive oil in a skillet over medium heat.
2. Add the ground pork and cook for 8-10 minutes, breaking into crumbles and stirring occasionally.
3. Add the salt, black pepper, thyme, sage, onion powder, cayenne pepper, red pepper flakes and maple syrup.
4. Mix to combine and cook for another minute or two.
5. Remove from the heat and set aside.
6. To make the crepes, in a bowl sift together the coconut flour, arrowroot flour, baking powder and salt and set aside.
7. In another bowl place the eggs and almond milk and whisk to combine.
8. Add in the coconut flour mixture and whisk to combine.
9. Let the batter sit for 5-10 minutes so it can thicken.
10. Preheat an 8 inch skillet over medium heat.
11. Lightly grease with olive oil.
12. Pour 3 tbsp of batter into the pan.
13. Swirl the pan so the bottom is evenly coated.
14. Cook for 2-3 minutes or until the top begins to appear dry and the edges start to brown, then flip carefully using a spatula.
15. Cook for another 1-2 minutes and then transfer to a serving plate.
16. Repeat the process to use the rest of the batter.
17. To assemble, place a crepe on a plate. Put some homemade sausage on one half of the crepe and sprinkle with chopped tomatoes. Top with a fried egg.
18. Fold 3 sides of the crepe inwards to form a half-closed, half-open pocket and serve.

Nutritional Information:

Calories 354 kcal |Potassium 487.7 mg |Vitamin A 108.3 µg |Vitamin C 2 mg |Folic Acid (B9) 30.4 µg |Sodium 511.3 mg

SNACKS:

Apple and Almond Butter Bites: These paleo-friendly apple and almond butter bites are easy to eat (no silverware required). Choose your apple and nut butter of choice and have some fun with toppings, like nuts or shredded coconut. For a lighter snack, halve the serving size. Per serving: 476 cal, 24 g fat (16 g sat), 66 g carbs, 50 g sugar, 132 mg sodium, 9.9 g fiber, 4.5 g protein.

Day 18

BREAKFAST: PALEO COD PICCATA

Ingredients

- 1 lb. cod fillets
- 1/3 cup almond flour
- 1/2 tsp salt
- 2-3 tbsp extra virgin olive oil
- 2 tbsp grapeseed oil, divided
- 3/4 cup chicken stock
- 3 tbsp lemon juice
- 1/4 cup capers, drained
- 2 tbsp fresh parsley, chopped

Preparations:

1. Stir the almond flour and salt together in a shallow bowl. Rinse off the fish and pat dry with a paper towel. Dredge the fish in the almond flour mixture to coat.
2. Heat enough olive oil to coat the bottom of a large skillet over medium-high heat along with one tablespoon grapeseed oil. Working in batches, add the cod and cook for 2-3 minutes per side to brown. Remove to a plate and set aside.
3. Add the chicken stock, lemon juice, and capers to the same skillet and scrape any browned bits off the bottom. Simmer to reduce the sauce by almost half. Remove from heat and stir in the remaining tablespoon of grapeseed oil.
4. To serve, divide the cod onto plates, drizzle with the sauce, and sprinkle with parsley.

Nutritional Information:

Calories 303 kcal | Potassium 607.9 mg | Vitamin A 22.6 μg | Vitamin C 8.1 mg | Folic Acid (B9) 16.8 μg | Sodium 470.8 mg

LUNCH: PALEO CROCK POT CHILI

Ingredients:

- 2 lbs. ground beef
- 1 medium onion, diced
- 4 cloves garlic, minced
- 1 red bell pepper, diced
- 1 green bell pepper, diced
- 3 stalks celery, diced
- 1 tomato, diced
- 1/4 cup diced green chilies
- 28 oz. can crushed tomatoes
- 15 oz. can tomato sauce
- 2 tbsp chili powder
- 1 tbsp oregano
- 1/2 tbsp basil
- 1/2 tbsp cumin
- 1/2 tbsp adobo sauce
- 1 tsp salt
- 1 tsp pepper
- 1/2 tsp cayenne

Preparations:

1. In a large skillet, sauté the onions and garlic over medium heat. Add in the ground beef and cook until browned. Drain the excess fat and then transfer the meat mixture to the crock pot.
2. Add in the bell peppers, celery, and diced tomato. Top with remaining ingredients and spices and stir everything together. Cook on low for 6-7 hours. Serve warm.

Nutritional Information:

Calories 367 kcal | Potassium 991.8 mg | Vitamin A 99.1 μg | Vitamin C 59.1 mg | Folic Acid (B9) 48 μg | Sodium 814.7 mg

DINNER: PALEO CROCK POT PULLED PORK

Ingredients:

- 3 lb. pork butt
- Salt and pepper
- 1 large yellow onion
- 4 chipotle peppers in adobo sauce and 3 tbsp sauce
- 1/2 cup Paleo Barbecue sauce
- 2 1/2 cups beef broth

Preparations:

1. Chop the onion into quarters and then layer into the bottom of the crock pot. Trim the pork butt of any excess fat and cut into 4-5 pieces. Season well with salt and pepper and lay on top of the onions. Add the peppers and adobo sauce, barbeque sauce, and broth. Cover and cook on low for 8-8.5 hours, until the pork is tender and easy to shred with a fork.
2. Remove the pork from the crock pot and shred. Set into a bowl. Strain the juices remaining in the crockpot through cheesecloth or a tea towel and add enough back to the shredded pork to coat.

Nutritional Information:

Calories 374 kcal | Potassium 829.5 mg | Vitamin A 222.8 µg | Vitamin C 26.3 mg | Folic Acid (B9) 9.2 µg | Sodium 864.9 mg

SNACKS:

Cauliflower Hummus Paleo + Low Carb: This cauliflower hummus is rich and creamy but low in carbs and perfectly paleo approved. It uses tahini, lemon, and smoked paprika for a flavorful dip with a spicy kick—and it tastes great as a filling for lettuce cups, or as a dip with veggie crudité. Per serving: 119 cal, 10.9 g fat (4.8 g sat), 4.8 g carbs, 1.1 g sugar, 1.8 g fiber, 2.3 g protein.

Day 19

BREAKFAST: SHRIMP & GRITS

Ingredients:

For the shrimp

- 15 pieces raw shrimp, shelled and de-veined
- 3 tbsp extra virgin olive oil
- 6 garlic cloves minced, divided
- Zest from one lemon
- 2 tsp dried oregano, divided
- 2 slices bacon
- 1/2 large onion, diced
- 2 tbsp butter
- 1 tbsp white wine vinegar
- 1 tsp red pepper flakes
- 1 tbsp lemon juice
- 1 tbsp chopped fresh oregano
- Salt and freshly ground black pepper, to taste

For the grits

- 1 large head of cauliflower, cut into florets
- 1/4 cup almond milk
- 4 garlic cloves, minced
- 1 tbsp ghee or butter
- 1/4 tsp cayenne pepper
- Salt and pepper, to taste

Preparations:

1. In a medium bowl mix together the olive oil, 2 cloves of garlic, lemon zest, and 1 teaspoon dried oregano. Place shrimp in the bowl and marinate for 1-3 hours.
2. Place a couple inches of water in a large pot. Once water is boiling, place steamer insert and then cauliflower florets into the pot and cover. Steam for 12-14 minutes, until completely tender. Drain and return cauliflower to pot.
3. Add the milk, ghee, and garlic to the cauliflower. Using an immersion blender, combine ingredients. The cauliflower should be fairly thick to resemble the consistency of grits.
4. Season with salt and pepper to taste.

5. Cook the bacon in a large skillet over medium heat until crispy. Reserving the bacon fat in the pan, set the bacon aside to cool and break into pieces.
6. Add the butter to the bacon fat in the pan and melt. Add the onion and sauté for 4-5 minutes until softened. Add in the remaining 4 garlic cloves, dried oregano, and the red pepper flakes. Sauté for 1-2 minutes, stirring frequently.
7. Stir in the white wine vinegar, and then add the shrimp. Cook, stirring frequently, until the shrimp are cooked through, 3-4 minutes. Remove from heat and stir in the lemon juice. Season with salt and pepper. Serve shrimp and onions over grits, with bacon and fresh oregano for garnish.

Nutritional Information:

Calories 334 kcal | Potassium 837.4 mg | Vitamin A 103.2 µg | Vitamin C 114.5 mg | Folic Acid (B9) 136.6 µg | Sodium 777.8 mg

LUNCH: PALEO TURKEY PESTO MEATBALLS

Ingredients:

- 2 lbs. ground turkey
- 1/2 cup almond flour
- 1/2 cup pesto
- 2 egg whites
- 1/2 tsp salt
- 1/4 tsp freshly ground pepper

Preparations:

1. Preheat the oven to 375 degrees F. Line a baking sheet with aluminum foil and then place a wire cooling rack on top of the baking sheet. Coat the wire rack well with coconut oil spray.
2. In a large bowl, mix together all of the ingredients. Roll the mixture into small balls using your hands and place on the wire rack. Bake for 20-25 minutes until cooked through.

Nutritional Information:

Calories 303 kcal |Potassium 382.4 mg |Vitamin A 109.9 µg |Vitamin C 5.7 mg |Folic Acid (B9) 29.4 µg |Sodium 324.2 mg

DINNER: AIR FRYER CRISPY CHICKEN

Ingredients:

- 2 pounds chicken drumstick
- 1 cup almond flour
- 1 ½ cup unsweetened finely shredded coconut
- 3 eggs, beaten
- ½ tsp smoked paprika
- ½ tsp garlic powder
- ½ tsp cayenne pepper
- 1 tbsp olive oil
- salt, black pepper

Preparations:

1. Generously season the drumsticks with salt and black pepper.
2. In a shallow plate add the almond flour, smoked paprika, garlic powder, cayenne pepper and good pinch of salt and black pepper. Mix to combine.
3. Beat the eggs in a small bowl. Season with pinch of salt.
4. Place the shredded coconut in a shallow dish.
5. Dip each chicken drumstick in the eggs then dredge in the almond flour mixture.
6. Dip each drumstick into the eggs again, followed by the shredded coconut.
7. Place the drumsticks on a chopping board and brush with olive oil.
8. Preheat a Philips air fryer to 360°F.
9. Place the drumsticks in a single layer in the fry basket and insert into the air fryer.
10. Cook for 18 minutes. Remove the drumsticks from the basket.
11. Repeat this process with the remaining drumsticks.
12. Serve warm.

Nutritional Information:

Calories 364 kcal |Potassium 407.1 mg |Vitamin A 42.3 µg |Vitamin C 0.3 mg |Folic Acid (B9) 11.3 µg |Sodium 334 mg

SNACKS:

Crock Pot Chunky Monkey Paleo Trail Mix: This yummy paleo trail mix includes dried banana slices, chocolate chips, coconut flakes, and nuts—like cashews, walnuts, or almonds—for a sweet, decadent-tasting recipe that's actually really good for you. To lighten it up, use half a cup of chocolate chips. Per serving: 250-260 cal, 20.2 g carbs, 3.5 to 4 g sugar, 18.6 to 22 g fiber, 12.5 to 13 g protein.

Day 20

BREAKFAST: PALEO SWEDISH MEATBALLS

Ingredients

- 1 pound ground beef
- 1 pound ground pork
- 1 small onion, diced
- 2 egg yolks
- ¼ tsp ground allspice
- ¼ tsp ground nutmeg
- ½ tsp salt
- ¼ tsp black pepper
- For the gravy
- 2 tbsp ghee
- 3 tbsp arrowroot flour
- 1 ½ cup hot beef broth
- ½ cup coconut milk, warmed
- 2 tablespoons chopped fresh parsley leaves

Preparations:

1. Add pork, beef, egg yolk, onion, nutmeg, allspice, salt and black pepper in a large bowl.
2. Mix to combine.
3. Shape into 1" balls.
4. Arrange meatballs in slow cooker.

5. In a skillet heat ghee over medium heat.
6. Add arrowroot flour and stir until smooth.
7. Add beef broth and coconut milk, whisking continuously until smooth.
8. Cook for 3-5 minutes.
9. Season to taste with salt and black pepper.
10. Pour sauce over meatballs, cover with a lid and cook for 4 hours on low.

Nutritional Information:

Calories 762 kcal | Potassium 908.9 mg | Vitamin A 94.3 µg | Vitamin C 5 mg | Folic Acid (B9) 36 µg | Sodium 616.3 mg

LUNCH: PALEO TORTILLA CHIPS

Ingredients:

- 1 cup almond flour
- 1 egg white
- 1/2 tsp salt
- 1/2 tsp chili powder
- 1/2 tsp garlic powder
- 1/2 tsp cumin
- 1/4 tsp onion powder
- 1/4 tsp paprika

Preparations:

1. Preheat the oven to 325 degrees F. In a large bowl, combine all of the ingredients together until they form an even dough.
2. Roll out the dough between two pieces of parchment paper, as thinly as possible. Remove the top layer of parchment paper. Cut the dough into desired shapes for chips.
3. Move the dough, with the parchment paper, onto a baking sheet. Bake for 11-13 minutes, until golden brown. Remove from the oven and let cool 5 minutes. Use a spatula to remove the chips from the paper. Serve with guacamole or salsa.

Nutritional Information:

Calories 171 kcal | Potassium 235.4 mg | Vitamin A 8.7 µg | Vitamin C 0.1 mg | Folic Acid (B9) 0.7 µg | Sodium 83.5 mg

DINNER: LEGENDARY GLUTEN-FREE BLUEBERRY CRISP

Ingredients:

- 2 pints fresh blueberries
- Juice of 1 lemon
- 1 cup almond flour
- 1/2 cup slivered almonds
- 1/4 cup coconut oil, melted
- 2 tbsp maple syrup
- 1 tsp cinnamon
- 1/8 tsp salt
- Pinch of nutmeg

Preparations:

1. Preheat the oven to 375 degrees F. In a small bowl, toss the blueberries with the lemon juice. Divide between six ramekin dishes.
2. Using the same bowl, mix together the remaining ingredients until combined. Spoon the almond crumble over the blueberries. Bake for 30-35 minutes, until bubbly and golden brown. Let cool slightly before serving.

Nutritional Information:

Calories 317 kcal | Potassium 307.3 mg | Vitamin A 3.1 µg | Vitamin C 14.7 mg | Folic Acid (B9) 11 µg | Sodium 50.9 mg

SNACKS:

Healthy Lemon Bars (gluten-free, dairy free & paleo): These lemon bars are tasty and decadent, but they're under 200 calories each. They're also made with healthier ingredients than the classic recipe—like almond flour, honey, and coconut oil. The crust is nice and crispy and the lemon filling is super-rich and creamy. Per serving: 189 cal, 11.5 g fat (4.9 g sat), 18.9 g carbs, 15.2 g sugar, 1.5 g fiber, 4.9 g protein.

BREAKFAST: SALMON STUFFED AVOCADOS

Ingredients:

- 6 oz can wild caught salmon drained
- 1/4 cup onion diced
- 2 tablespoon minced pimentos
- 1 tablespoon olive oil
- 1 tablespoon chopped fresh parsley
- Juice of 1 lemon
- 2 mini avocados

Preparations:

1. Combine the salmon, onion, pimentos, olive oil, parsley, and lemon juice in a small bowl. Mix well.
2. When ready to serve, cut the avocados in half and remove the pit. Fill the avocado halves with the salmon mixture right before serving.

Nutritional Information:

Calories: 249.6 |Total Fat: 19.3 g |Dietary Fiber: 5.9 g |Saturated Fat: 3.7 g

LUNCH: PALEO CARROT CAKE CUPCAKES

Ingredients:

- 3 large carrots
- 4-5 pitted Medjool dates
- 3 eggs
- 1/4 cup honey
- 2 tbsp coconut oil, melted
- 1 1/2 cups almond flour
- 2 tsp cinnamon
- 1/2 tsp salt
- 1/2 tsp baking soda

- 1/2 tsp nutmeg
- 1 cup walnuts, finely chopped

For the frosting:

- 1 14-oz. can coconut milk, chilled
- 1 tsp honey
- 1/2 tsp cinnamon
- 1/2 tsp vanilla extract
- Pinch of ground cloves

Preparations:

1. Preheat the oven to 325 degrees F. Line a muffin tin with cups. Coarsely chop the carrots and dates and place in a food processor. Pulse until finely chopped. In a large bowl, whisk together the eggs, honey, and coconut oil. Add the carrots and dates and stir well.
2. In a separate bowl, stir together the almond flour, cinnamon, salt, baking soda, and nutmeg. Mix the dry ingredients into the wet ingredients and stir to combine. Fold in the chopped walnuts.
3. Divide the batter equally among the muffin cups, filling each cup about 3/4 of the way full. Bake for 20-25 minutes, or until a toothpick inserted into the center comes out clean. Let cool for 5 minutes, and then transfer to a wire rack to cool completely.
4. To make the frosting, blend together the chilled coconut cream (spooned from the top of the can), honey, cinnamon, vanilla, and ground cloves in a food processor until completely combined. Spread over the cooled cupcakes.

Nutritional Information:

Calories 383.5 |Total Fat 34.2 g |Saturated Fat 19.3 g |Polyunsaturated Fat 3.7 g |Monounsaturated Fat 7.0 g |Cholesterol 118.3 mg |Sodium 304.0 mg

|Potassium 190.4 mg |Total Carbohydrate 17.4 g |Dietary Fiber 7.9 g |Sugars 5.7 g |Protein 9.6 g

DINNER: REPEATING THE PALEO CROCK POT PULLED PORK

Ingredients:

- 3 lb. pork butt
- Salt and pepper
- 1 large yellow onion
- 4 chipotle peppers in adobo sauce and 3 tbsp sauce
- 1/2 cup Paleo Barbecue sauce
- 2 1/2 cups beef broth

Preparations:

1. Chop the onion into quarters and then layer into the bottom of the crock pot. Trim the pork butt of any excess fat and cut into 4-5 pieces. Season well with salt and pepper and lay on top of the onions. Add the peppers and adobo sauce, barbeque sauce, and broth. Cover and cook on low for 8-8.5 hours, until the pork is tender and easy to shred with a fork.
2. Remove the pork from the crock pot and shred. Set into a bowl. Strain the juices remaining in the crockpot through cheesecloth or a tea towel and add enough back to the shredded pork to coat.

Nutritional Information:

Calories 374 kcal |Potassium 829.5 mg |Vitamin A 222.8 µg |Vitamin C 26.3 mg |Folic Acid (B9) 9.2 µg |Sodium 864.9 mg

SNACKS:

Turmeric Stove Top Paleo Granola: This easy, 15-minute granola recipe is packed with anti-inflammatory spices, like turmeric and cinnamon, and it has a wonderful balance of sweet, spicy, and savory. Each snack serving is under 200 calories, and it has lots of good fats and protein from the coconut, seeds, and nuts. For a more substantial snack, add to a plain Greek yogurt. Per serving: 191 cal, 16 g fat (8 g sat), 9 g carbs, 8 g sugar, 6 mg sodium, 3 g fiber, 3 g protein

The effectiveness of the paleo diet is very popular, and its benefits are interesting! In addition to helping you lose weight, this diet is ideal for feeling fit, but also for gaining muscle mass. However, keep in mind that this slimming program is restrictive in that it prohibits many foods. Another disadvantage: it can lead to nutritional deficiencies due to the absence of certain foods such as dairy products. We must be careful and consume a large number of fruits and vegetables to fill these gaps. Moreover, it is not suitable for everyone; do not forget to ask a professional his opinion. Only he can tell you whether or not the Paleo diet is right for you.

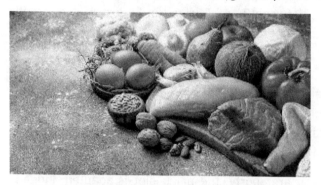

But despite its restrictive side, the paleo diet brings a feeling of satiety because of its richness in proteins and fibers; an interesting point that allows you to be full and not feel a feeling of hunger during his diet. Another plus point: the number of meals and portions depend on each one. There is no taxation.

So is the paleo diet a good or bad idea? Absolutely, you can find this diet effective for losing weight quickly. However, some of its principles can be adopted to lose weight, but do not fall into the extreme risk of suffering its disadvantages.

The virtues of the paleo diet on health, what are they?

The Paleolithic diet is based on a healthy and natural diet. In addition to helping you eliminate your extra pounds, this slimming method is also beneficial to gain muscle mass and to regain better health and fitness.

Regarding weight loss, the Paleo diet removes processed foods, already prepared dishes and starchy foods; foods that cause weight gain. During this diet, the feeling of satiety is also filled by proteins derived from vegetables and lean meats. Thanks to the satiating effect of these foods, you will not be hungry, and you will not be tempted to nibble.

The fibers contained in the Paleolithic diet are in turn beneficial for the intestinal transit and to promote digestion. This diet also helps prevent the development of cardiovascular disease through the consumption of omega-3-rich oilseeds.

The paleo diet is a slimming program that ensures a mild and not brutal weight loss: on average, between 3 and 5 kilos can be lost in one month, provided you consume the right foods.

Precautions to take

If you want to feel better, following the principles of the paleo diet is a good idea. However, its restrictive side does not make it a diet suitable for everyone. This is why it is important to consult your doctor before putting it in place.

On the other hand, if you are sporty, the paleo diet is adapted. Indeed, physical exercise works in synergy with this slimming program to reduce fat and increase muscle. Following the Paleolithic diet is also effective for increasing performance and being more energetic.

100% natural, the Paleolithic diet is a satiating and effective slimming program that leads to interesting weight loss and better shape. With the paleo diet, you will adopt a natural diet and good for health: more dishes already prepared and more fast food. You will eat fruits, vegetables, and meat! In contrast, the Paleo diet excludes many food categories such as dairy products. It is, therefore, necessary to consume fruits and vegetables in sufficient quantity to avoid suffering from nutritional deficiencies.

The paleo diet is also a method that requires motivation. In fact, at the same time frustrating and monotonous, this diet can be difficult to follow and can be a source of social isolation. To follow it well and to keep it, you have to be determined!

If you feel ready to eat in the same way as our ancestors, all you have to do is set up the Paleolithic diet just for 3 weeks and experience the perfect way to lose weight and avoid obesity!

KINDLY NOTE:

Hope you enjoy the inspired and fun recipes featured in this book. However, the information in this book is not responsible for the outcome of any recipe you try from this book. You may not achieve desired results due to variations in elements such as ingredients, cooking temperatures, typos, errors, omissions, or individual cooking ability. You should always use your best judgment when cooking with raw ingredients such as eggs, chicken, or seafood and seek expert advice before beginning if you are unsure. You should always take care when using sharp knives or other cooking implements. To ensure the safety of yourself and others, be aware of heated cooking surfaces while cooking. Please review all ingredients before trying a recipe to be fully aware of the presence of substances which might cause an adverse reaction in some consumers. Recipes available in this book may not have been formally tested, and this book does not provide any assurances nor accept any responsibility or liability with regard to their originality, quality, nutritional value, or safety.

And also I am not a health care practitioner. All the information you read on recipes is purely for informational and educational purposes. Information is not intended to treat, cure or prevent any disease. Statements within this book have not been approved, meaning the Food and Drug Administration has not evaluated information and statements regarding health claims. All information is solely my personal experiences and opinions and should not be interpreted as an attempt to offer a medical opinion as the writer of this book is not responsible for any adverse reactions, effects, or consequences resulting from the use of any recipes or suggestions herein or procedures undertaken hereafter. If you have questions about food, diet, nutrition, natural remedies or holistic health, please do your research and consult with your health care practitioner to adjust to the right amount of calories, once that can be achieved you can modify each recipe as you require. If you are pregnant, nursing, have a medical condition or are taking any medications, please consult your health care practitioner before making any changes to your diet or supplement regimen.

You can also calculate the amount of calories you need with the following websites:

- https://www.myfitnesspal.com
- https://www.loseit.com
- https://www.fatsecret.com
- https://cronometer.com
- https://www.sparkpeople.com
- https://www.healthline.com/nutrition/how-many-calories-per-day
- https://www.calculator.net/calorie-calculator.html
- https://www.freedieting.com/calorie-calculator

Chapter Sixteen
Paleo Diet: The Right Diet for Athletes

More and more people interested in the Paleolithic diet to maintain health. Is this diet compatible with sports performance?

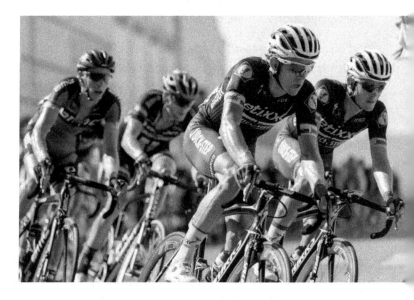

In recent years, the paleo diet derived from the Paleolithic word, which takes the principles of feeding our ancestors, returns to the forefront. But think about it: despite its name, it's not just a temporary dietary measure designed to make you lose those extra pounds. Above all, it is a way of life that is long-term, allowing people to eat healthier, lose extra pounds, and prevent many of the chronic diseases of our time, such as obesity and stroke, and diabetes. It, therefore, calls for a radical and sustainable transformation of our diet, which is richer in protein, good lipids, and unprocessed vegetables. In other words,

So what are the main principles of the paleo diet? And how to integrate it effectively and sustainably into one's lifestyle, even as the modern diet has significantly changed our eating habits?

This diet brings undeniable advantages. Firstly, the absence of foods with a high glycemic index favors the use of fats and limits weight gain, two effects that are particularly beneficial for endurance athletes. Moreover, the alkalizing character of this diet is interesting because of its protective role of bone capital and the limitation of muscle wasting, which is important for the athlete. On the other hand, the reduction of allergenic foods such as gluten and dairy products helps protect the digestive system which limits inflammatory and autoimmune diseases. This protective role of the digestive system is useful to the athlete because intensive sports practice (especially running) attacks the digestive system. In addition, it could help to limit too frequent digestive disorders to the effort. The richness of omega 3 is obviously another benefit of this food model especially when we know the benefits of omega 3 in endurance athletes (improvement of the use of lipids: s effort, limitation of excessive inflammatory phenomena especially). However, this diet will not be easily compatible with the practice of intensive endurance sports.

The Paleo diet is an old concept, but it is very interesting. Unfortunately, putting it into practice can be difficult: for example, the fat quality of meat from animals is not the same as at the time, with the consequences of health that we know. Nevertheless, some principles are very interesting for the health of many people: the suppression of cereals, the abundance of plants and the increase in omega-3 intakes are fundamental elements of an anti-inflammatory diet that can help maintain a healthy lifestyle. Good bone mass, to avoid the onset of diabetes and probably to reduce the symptoms of most diseases with chronic inflammation or certain autoimmune diseases, particularly thinking of ankylosing spondylitis or rheumatoid arthritis. Nevertheless, this diet is not suitable for everyone.

Simple, healthy, and natural, hunter-gatherer feeding also helps eliminate all toxins from the body, battling potential disrupters and improving the balance of the intestinal flora. The body thus regenerated starts to work better, and this is felt with a significant improvement in energy levels and effective weight loss, especially bad fats.

Above all, it must be realized that the intensive practice of an endurance sport is not "paleo." For the occasional endurance athlete, this type of diet may be suitable as long as you eat a lot of vegetables and fruits. While for the endurance athlete more intensive, it will be difficult with this diet to have a sufficient carbohydrate ration. However, we can adapt the diet by providing enough carbohydrate while trying to reduce their impact on insulin. For this, we can eat foods richer in carbohydrates but low glycemic index (legumes, sweet potatoes, fruits, possibly unrefined cereals for those who tolerate them ...). In addition, we will seek to use the " metabolic windows talking about taking advantage of the times when carbohydrate ingestion will be fully profitable. It should be known that just after a sufficiently intense effort, the muscle cells have worked will quickly absorb carbohydrates and that without insulin. This both limits insulin secretion and optimizes carbohydrate intake by providing carbohydrates that will only be used to replenish glycogen stores used during exercise. This makes it possible to optimize muscular functioning while limiting fat gain.

The Paleo diet will be compatible with most strength sports, but there will be large individual variations on the impact in terms of physical development and performance. We are all genetically different, and some people use carbohydrates better to provide energy than others. For this group, the Paleo diet will not allow such a rapid progression when carbohydrate intake is higher and performance may be reduced. In addition, the Paleo diet does not allow a "mass gain" specific to bodybuilding, during which insulin levels must be high, which is difficult with this ancestral diet. But having said that, "mass gaining" is far from being a good technique for health.

The endurance sportsman will often be interested in approaching (without excess). In the endurance sportsman "performer" during intensive training, it is possible to consider departing from the "paleo" diet during sports and just after to find a "paleo" diet for the rest of the time. In this same endurance sportsman "performer," it is possible to get as close as possible to the "paleo" diet during rest and recovery phases at the end of the season in order to "reprogram" his cells for better use of lipids which will be beneficial for endurance. The Paleo model could be useful for the endurance athlete who does not "perform" and does not perform too much intensity, always with the same aim of improving the use of lipids. Also, this could be particularly useful for the athlete who is looking to lose weight because it promotes fat loss while maintaining muscle mass.

Absolutely, as part of a weight loss for a strength athlete, the Paleo diet concentrates all the assets necessary for success: good protein intake, significant amounts of fat, lots of vegetables and low glycemic index low carbohydrates. In muscle mass gain if you try to limit fat gain, the Paleo diet is also very effective, especially for people whose body uses carbohydrates badly.

Before you train, you could, for example, eat raspberries or blackberries that contain a lot of fiber and reduce insulin rises. The blueberries will also make a great snack because they contain lots of antioxidants. A handful of nuts (almonds, pistachios, walnuts) will also be an excellent snack as it is one of the best sources of monounsaturated fats that are excellent for the heart.

It is now up to you to opt for this type of training by running in a perfect match with your Paleo diet! Less monotonous than your usual jogging this type of session will make you progress fast and will make you more dry and vigorous, but do not forget the fundamentals: hydration and progressivity.

Chapter Seventeen
Budget Secrets for A Paleo Diet Grocery List

The essence of a paleo diet is to eat simply as our hunter-gatherer ancestors did. Therefore, you should avoid industrially processed foods, refined foods, junk foods, sugary drinks, carbonated soft drinks, etc.

In fact, all the foods mentioned above occupy a huge percentage of grocery list spending!

But below you will find out how easy it is in a paleo diet to save unnecessary money spent on buying these expensive and unhealthy foods.

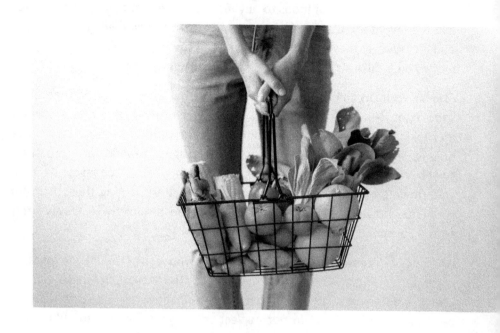

How to Save On Food

Below are suggestions that will help you save money on groceries to buy in a paleo diet.

Plan ahead for the list of foods to buy: Before you go shopping, a simple idea like the inventory of foods to buy to fill the pantry will help you keep your budget. Weekly meal planning and creating a shopping list will help save money on food and cooking gas.

Choose Your Organic Product: Studies reveal that some fruits and vegetables should not be bought in large markets because of their wealth of pesticides and toxic residues. While the products you can find in organic stores like onions, eggplants, broccoli, cabbage, asparagus, cauliflower, tomatoes, sweet potatoes, avocado, pineapple, mango, kiwi, papaya, banana, watermelon, etc. are some of the products that are lacking these harmful elements. However, it is essential to wash the product well, always and before consuming it.

Growing A Vegetable Garden: For those who can, creating an organic vegetable garden at home is the cheapest way to consume organic products. This guarantees not only fresh products but above all products without pesticide residues. Also, do not neglect the physical activity to cultivate a vegetable garden that positively affects health. For those who also own a large yard, they can exaggerate by raising animals such as chickens that in addition to providing fertilizer for the garden, can also produce organic eggs.

Local Market: The local market could be a good place to buy grass-fed meat and organic eggs at a lower price. Visiting the farmer's market, at the end of the day, in the afternoon it will surely be a very good profit, as farmers tend to s-sell their products to avoid making them rot. This translates into great offers and good business, especially for meat.

Choosing seasonal foods: Consuming seasonal foods is a great way to save money. They can also be purchased in bulk and frozen for later consumption.

Fishing or Hunting: Those who hunt and or fish as a hobby can benefit greatly both from a playful and an economic point of view. Getting food like our ancestors is certainly an added value for what we eat

Visits to agri-tourisms or orchards: A visit to the orchard or the agricultural agri-tourism will be able to give the joy of collecting berries or picking fresh apples. This will entail great economic savings and will benefit from freshly harvested fruit/vegetables at a lower cost than stores. Since the products are specifically harvested by hand, the preservation capacity, taste, and nutrition of the product are intact over a long period of time, unlike the store where the dubious origin of the products do not guarantee their durability.

Avoid wasting food: Learning to cook and use the ingredients available in the kitchen makes preparing dinner less expensive and more fun. This obviously becomes simpler when the weekly requirement is planned in advance.

Expensive Diet?

The Paleo diet may seem expensive but try replacing a shopping cart that was previously filled with junk foods, pre-cooked foods and treated with healthy foods like nuts and fruit.

It should also be remembered following some Paleolithic advice that greater physical activity and a less sedentary life must be done. This, in turn, must be seen as a means to save money, avoiding taking the car to reach nearby destinations, favoring the use of the bicycle or one's legs for a nice walk in the open air.

If the paleo diet focuses on fresh produce, having a strong grocery store (longer shelf life products) will make your life a lot easier, and help you out the day you forget to shop.

On the other hand, here is a list of foods you should always have at home if you follow the paleo diet.

Spices, herbs, condiments

Condiments play a key role in our diet, as they make the difference between a banal dish and an excellent dining experience.

- Mustard
- Pickles
- Herbs and spices: Have heaps.

A Habit to Take: when you go through the herbs & spices section of your supermarket, do not think and grab the first mill that comes to hand. As you build up a good stock, you keep it at hand when cooking (let yourself be inspired by the moment).

Also, don't forget the first option which is to consider growing on your balcony or in your garden small plants of thyme, parsley, mint, etc. This requires almost no maintenance, and the taste of fresh herbs is unparalleled.

Salt Pepper: Preserves

- It is always good to have some preserves in front of you, to decorate a salad, or go on a picnic.
- Artichoke hearts
- Bamboo shoots
- Tuna inbox
- Canned sardines/mackerel (watch out for vegetable oils, prefer preparations with olive oil)
- Canned cod liver (an excellent source of omega-3, to be consumed in salads)

Frozen: Frozen products are an excellent solution for troubleshooting when you run out of fresh produce (always favor the expense).

- Minced meat
- Fish fillets (salmon, trout)
- Shrimp
- Frozen vegetables (fried various, spinach, cauliflower, mushrooms, etc.)
- The mix of red fruits

For The Kitchen: These are the recurring ingredients in Paleo recipes, or you'll need to cook on a daily basis.

- Duck or goose fat
- Tomato puree (100% tomato)
- Lean cocoa powder (100% cocoa)
- Coconut milk (beware of additives)
- Recalled coconut
- Coconut flour
- Almond powder
- Olive oil
- Coconut oil
- Chicken broth

- Vinegar

Other

In this part, the unclassifiable.

- Almonds / cashews / walnuts / hazelnuts / etc. Always take fresh nuts (avoid salty/roasted versions)
- Almond butter
- Olives (to prepare tapenade for example) or aperitif time
- Dried fruits: apricots, prunes, dates, figs, etc.

Once again, following the paleo diet means eating fresh foods: meats, fish, eggs, vegetables, and fruits, not to mention the market herbs. Hence, it's up to you now.

Chapter Eighteen
Preventing Illness with Paleo Diet Grocery List

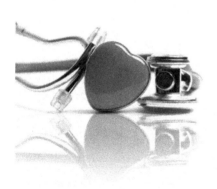

When we go into the paleo, we often tend to avoid gray areas and to classify food in two categories: "good" and "bad." Bread? Wrong. Hot dog? Wrong. Broccoli? Good. Steak? Good. It helps not to break your head when you are grocery shopping, but the food industry often finds a way to sabotage our food and sometimes you have to take the time to get down to things in more detail. Here is a list of foods that are technically paleo, but want to avoid as much as possible.

- **Poor Quality Olive Oil**

Since being recognized as a staple of the Mediterranean diet, the diet typically known as excellent for health, olive oil has gained tremendous popularity. Unfortunately, this popularity has a price: corruption in the industry is very high. For example, in some countries, much of the production is controlled by mafia organizations, and a 2011 survey showed that 80% of "extra-virgin" oils are cut with oils of lower quality. Sometimes it's olive oil extracted more industrially, or sometimes it's just canola oil or soybean oil.

Here is a list of what you can look for when you buy an olive oil:

The mention extra-virgin and cold pressed. It may be wrong, but it's better than buying olive oil that has been hot-extracted and with industrial solvents.

An opaque bottle. If the bottle is transparent, the antioxidants in the oil will degrade because of the light. A producer who has his olive oil at heart will be careful to protect it with a quality bottle.

Harvest date and an expiration date. It assures you that the oil is not a mixture of different oils, some of which might be shady.

A strong olive taste. Olive oil that tastes nothing is usually more refined and is more likely to be contaminated with a neutral oil such as canola oil.

- **Palm Oil**

Palm oil has been used by humans for millennia and can be excellent for your health. It is nourishing, and it is very rich in carotenoids when it is extracted correctly. Unfortunately, most of what is on the market are very processed (refined, bleached, deodorized) and no longer contains antioxidants. Moreover, and this is a big problem; most of the palm oil found on the market is the product of massive deforestation. It is, among other things, the main cause of the disappearance of orangutan habitats in Indonesia. Some palm oils are sustainably produced, but they are hard to find, and their taste is good enough to make it worthwhile. Unrefined palm oil has a rich orange color, a sign that it contains carotenoids.

- **Coconut Milk with Shady Ingredients**

As a big fan of coconut in general. It's nourishing, it's versatile, it's delicious, and it's good for your health. One often use coconut milk in recipes or smoothies and coffee. You need to be very selective when you buy because companies tend to put several processed ingredients so that the texture remains uniform. If the list of ingredients contains anything other than coconut and water, then stay away.

When you buy coconut milk make sure you mainly buy the right brand that contains coconut and water, is reasonably priced and has a delicious taste.

- **Roasted Walnuts in Oil**

Nuts are a food of choice for people who go paleo: they are nutritious, they keep well, they are excellent for health, they are rich in protein and cut hunger and, for people who pay attention they are very low in carbohydrates. The major problem is that they are often roasted in vegetable oil, such as soybean oil or canola oil, highly processed oils that we want to avoid at all costs.

What do we want to choose instead? Either dry roasted nuts or raw nuts roasted oneself. It can easily be found in specialized shops. No matter what nuts you buy, if the list of ingredients contains the term "vegetable oil," please stay away.

- **Commercial Honey**

Like olive oil, the commercial honey found on the shelves is very likely to be contaminated by several shady substances. Honey is the third most defunct food in the world, and you have to be wary of honey from the Asian market. Honey from China, for example, is often contaminated with noxious products banned in Canada and Europe and is often even mixed with cheaper sugar, such as corn syrup.

What do we buy instead? Fortunately, you can buy honey that comes directly from the honey house — guaranteed that it is of excellent quality with reasonable prices. Bonus: if you have children, take the opportunity to visit the facilities. Many honey producers have systems where the hive can be seen through transparent windows, and it is a great opportunity for a child to learn where the food comes from, and the importance of paying attention to wild spaces with flowers.

However, the main principle is simple: we can try to minimize the misdeeds of the modern world on our body by partially inspiring us in the way of life of our ancestors:

Have a good quality diet based on REAL foods and, if possible, organic and whole. Food that includes the consumption of vegetables and fruits of the season, meat (rather lean), fish, oilseeds, eggs, if this diet comes from local products it's even better.

- Take time to organize and cook ... and avoid prepared dishes.
- Minimize cooking and favor raw food: cooking tends to transform food and denature.
- Eat according to the needs and desires of your body without necessarily counting calories.
- Have regular physical activity and optimized for the human body.
- Spend a lot of time outdoors.

Conversely, the idea is also to avoid foods that did not exist a few thousand years ago. Indeed, the profound changes that have appeared in our diet with the massive consumption of industrial food, cereals, and dairy products would have resulted in a conflict with our original genes. This seems quite plausible since 10,000 years represent less than 1% of the evolutionary history of man.

Hence, we often buy "paleo" food with the best intentions, but we can be fooled by the food industry if we do not stay on our guard. Take the time to read the nutrition labels in preventing illness with Paleo Diet Grocery List!

Chapter Nineteen
When you Follow the Paleo Diet, You Can Also Enjoy Life

You are now familiar with "Paleo Diet" - and we have already written extensively from the beginning of this book. Eat the foods with which the human species has evolved, avoid those who have just appeared on our plates, it is consistent. But, beyond food, there are many ways to take inspiration from the evolution of our species, from what we know, to live in better health. Sleep, stress management, physical activity, our time is not lacking challenges. Of course, it is not possible to live today as in 8001 BC, but the man of the Paleolithic can be a source of inspiration to a better life. So let's see how you can also enjoy life with paleo diet today.

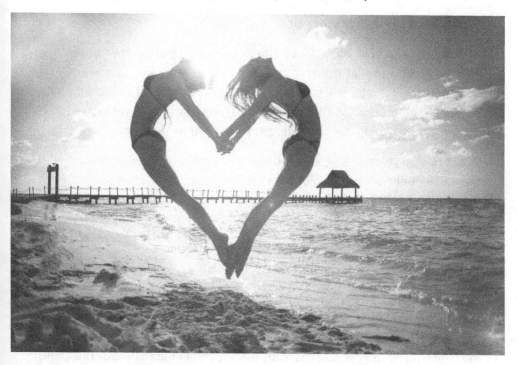

Better Sleep and Better Wake Up

One in three people has difficulty falling asleep. Among the causes, the increasing exposure, at night, to the blue light emitted by the screens. The body perceives this blue light as that of the day, as a signal that clearly says standing! The production of melatonin, the sleep hormone, is then reduced leaving our eyes wide open and the circadian rhythm disrupted.

Over 1 million years, this light signal was not a problem; it was associated with the daytime period. What solution, then? The extinction of all screens from sunset? Impossible in most cases.

Hence, technology has come to create hormonal chaos, and it also brings the antidote. Here are paleo technical solutions to bring us closer to a more archaic luminous environment, in which melatonin can increase gradually after sunset, as it should be:

The simplest solution, the installation of an application on your computers (PC / Mac) and on your iPhone (or Twilight for Android) that gradually filters the blue light from your screens from sunset, and in the middle of the night, there is no blue coming out of these screens. The most radical solution is to wear orange sunglasses at night to filter out this blue light. A guaranteed effect, and from all points of view.

After a 7- to 9-hour sleep - the length of time most adults need - waking up. Being woken up by a ring is stressful. Other solutions have been around for a long time, including dawn simulators. More recently, an app installed on your phone, will analyze the depth of your sleep and wake you up at the right time, when your sleep is the lightest. It works.

Settling in The Office, Paleo Way

11 am in the office. Sitting in front of a screen, 8 hours a day, has several significant negative effects, among which a reduced production of the fat-burning enzyme LPL (lipoprotein lipase), a decrease of the mineral density of the bones, an increase blood pressure and a decrease in the diameter of the arteries.

Let's go back to the origins: this position, for the human being, is not natural. What is natural is an alternation of walking, standing, and squatting. The resting position of our ancestors was squatting and not sitting. This being the case, for most of us, this position is unnatural and quickly becomes difficult to hold.

What to Do? Crouch On the Floor at The Office?

Less extreme but still far from the norm: the office upright. Better, the office placed above a treadmill (yes, it exists, and it's called a "treadmill desk"). More seriously, you have to alternate different positions.

Depending on where you work, you have alternatives to prolonged sitting. Getting up and taking a walk, or even a real break, every 45 minutes is a good start to mitigate the effects of sitting. Incidentally, it makes the work much more efficient. Doing some meetings while walking is often possible and again, more effective. And if you work from home with a laptop, it's easy to alternate between standing, back and sitting.

The Break

In "lunch break" there is a break, and there is lunch. Let's start with the break, following the previous point. Take advantage of this break to go for a walk, ideally in a park next door, otherwise just in the street, it is very paleo.

But to push the experience even further, walk barefoot. Oh no, this is wacky ideas! But is it possible? Not too much, in general. But then again, get technology help, it's the beauty of our time to use technology to live like in the Paleolithic era.

Paleo fashion is barefoot shoes, barefoot. Initially, we only found this kind of shoes with each insulated toe, as in a glove. This type of shoe perfectly fits the foot to simulate walking and running barefoot. But today, there are other more discreet options, and therefore more adapted to the context of the lunch break. These shoes have a very thin sole that allows you to feel the ground on which you walk.

The benefits? On another hand, there are simply benefits in walking. The human being walks from its origins, and the whole body is a machine to walk. Displacement on the back of an animal only appeared after agriculture, very recently in the history of the species.

Our species has evolved barefoot until a very recent past; our feet are designed for this. Defending thick soles to protect the joints, it's the same vein as defending sunscreen against the sun, the sun that accompanies humanity since its origins.

The Lunch

Not always easy, to have lunch outside, when one is fond of paleo. The Paleo's food base is to eat only foods that existed before the introduction of agriculture 10,000 years ago, with a few well-chosen exceptions. We feed on the food that has accompanied the evolution of the human species, validated by tens of thousands of generations. It's unbeatable. It eliminates all those appeared during the last millennia, including cereals, dairy products and of course industrial products, including vegetable oils.

This avoids, in particular, to create panic movements among the hormones. The elimination of refined flours and sugars, in particular, avoids regular flooding of insulin blood to eliminate these repeated peak blood sugar levels. That's where the difficulty comes from today. When all these recent food products are removed, what remains?

In order to have a paleo lunch, you have several options. The first is to do the impasse. Quite simply. In some contexts, especially traveling, there is not really a good option for healthy eating. In this case, do not eat lunch.

If you adopt a Paleo diet, cravings will gradually disappear. The glycemic caused by the peaks of sugar in the blood will no longer concern you. And your sensitivity to insulin will probably have increased, allowing you to tap into your fat reserves and hold until evening more easily. Multiple benefits, you have fasted, with all that it brings to the body, and you have consumed some of your fat stock.

Another option is to prepare your lunch the night before and bring it with you. And if you go to the restaurant anyway, choose it well. The sushi version is a good choice. Grill and vegetables, it's acceptable. The salad shop too, if you make the salad yourself with paleo ingredients, on a quinoa or lettuce base. Skip pasta, pizzas, quiches, fried products, sandwiches, and mysterious sauces. Not just for the reasons you already know, but also because it's made from totally non-paleo industrial products (refined flours and vegetable oils).

You can also cut the hunger by making you happy, with paleo snacks such as chocolate 90% or almonds, and with moderation. It's fat, but in the context of a paleo diet, we prefer this fat to sugary alternatives by far.

Back in The Office: Manage The Permanent Alert

In today's classic work environment, your desk phone rings and flashes. Your phone vibrates briefly to display a notification; the summary of each email is displayed for a few seconds at the bottom right of your computer; news briefs scroll. It's the permanent alert.

Even if, in the realm of reactivity, this mode of operation can today often seem inevitable, it is an aberration from the point of view of the evolution of our species.

The human body knows how to react to the alert. He knows how to react to stress. This mechanism is provided for survival purposes, to cope with situations of life and death, those where it is necessary to fight or to take the legs to his neck. A flow of adrenaline, cortisol and a whole host of other hormones is produced for that. The whole body mobilizes against the danger, the immune system pauses, some maintenance mechanisms stop.

The modern workstation generates an uninterrupted sequence of small stresses. And the human body has not yet adapted to these new sources of stress. The body is the amalgam between real danger and this ordinary everyday business. What made sense in an ancestral environment becomes completely inadequate today, and it is dangerous. To constantly activate the mechanisms of reaction to danger is to find ourselves too often in a state where the body does not respect its immune defense and its mechanisms of internal maintenance. And it is also taking the risk of gradually decreasing its sensitivity to these hormones, pushing the body to produce more and more, until exhaustion.

These sources of permanent stress are virtually impossible to eliminate today. Again, for the most part, we have neither the luxury nor the desire to go live as a hermit in the woods (although, sometimes). Put in place means to limit the impact of these new sources of stress. However, it is possible.

One of the most effective methods for this is to disable all notifications. Almost all. Disable notifications of new emails, personal and professional, disable notifications Facebook, WhatsApp, Twitter, do not receive real-time info, do not systematically answer calls. Maybe keep a channel to join if it's urgent: in some cases, the SMS. All these messages, then treat them in batches, once or twice a day.

Initially, you need to educate your personal and professional contacts, so that this new way of working is known: You can answer at a certain moment, but not immediately. With a dose of discipline, it works. The secondary benefit, efficiency increases with this newfound concentration, and the meetings become useful again when one learns to raise the eyes of his phone. Does the whole world get on alert because you are not responding in real time? No, believe me, in general, it adapts gradually to you. This is a key principle to reduce stress: do not let others manage your day. Easier said than done? Try a week, then adjust.

Do You Know?

It is always interesting to understand the context in which the human species has evolved, and to grasp the gap that separates this ancestral context from ours, today. Some dysfunctions come back: some hormonal responses, intended to be episodic, are solicited at an even higher frequency. These hormonal responses, which have become crazy, gradually weaken the body. Understanding this, and learning to reduce these simulations to regulate your hormonal flows better, is a fundamental approach to taking care of your health. It brings to the physiological mechanisms a context closer to the one in which we have evolved. So the paleo, today is possible with a little imagination, discipline, and information.

Chapter Twenty
Preventing and Treating Depression with the Paleo Diet

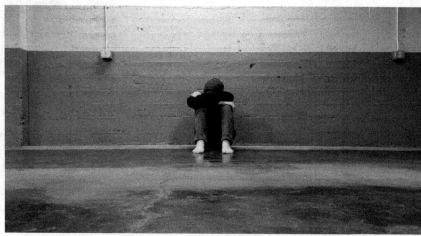

Depression is a chronic disease characterized by feelings of sadness and loneliness. According to WebMD, other symptoms include a loss of interest in activities that were once pleasant and a decrease in energy. A healthy diet, such as the Paleolithic diet can help reduce depressive symptoms thanks to the consumption of nutritiously healthy substances and thanks to the absence of processed and refined foods.

Depression in Women

According to research the rates of depression between the women who had followed a western diet, with those of women who had followed a traditional diet, made of vegetables, fruit, meat, fish and whole grains. The traditional diet is similar in its composition to that of the Paleolithic diet as it eliminates refined foods. Women who had followed a western diet of processed foods, sugar-rich products, and refined grains showed significantly higher rates of depression.

Mechanisms of Depression

Mechanisms of Depression include interruption of three fundamental systems - neurotransmitter metabolism, neuroendocrine function, and neuroplasticity. All these malfunctions are caused by slight but chronic inflammation. A Paleolithic diet can help fight depression by reducing inflammation.

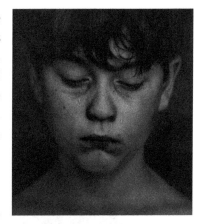

Omega-3 And Depression

Omega-3 fatty acids have been shown to be an effective treatment for depression. The Paleolithic diet includes natural sources of omega-3. Fish, especially varieties of cold water like salmon and mackerel are full of these nutritious fats. Green leafy vegetables, such as spinach and kale, are also good sources of omega-3. Game and beef raised and fattened with grass offer much more omega-3 fatty acids than domesticated animals, even partially bred with wheat. So the next time you feel a little down, think about goods before you stretch the embers for an unhealthy snack. Prepare Paleo snacks at home.

Chapter Twenty-One
Interesting Health Benefits of Going Paleo

The paleo diet is by far one of the most popular diets in recent years, alongside gluten-free diets and Detox diets. Most people imagine that nutrition programs like the paleo diet are the perfect way to lose weight, but it's a mistake! The paleo diet is not just an instrument to lose weight, and it's a whole new way of eating. Once you know the foods you can eat as a paleo

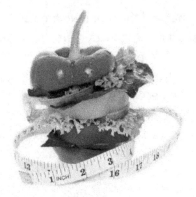

follower and master some recipes, you'll have a better understanding of what this nutritional approach is.

In nature, we would not be able to consume most of what we call cereals (spelled, barley, rice, buckwheat, etc.). In nature, we would find them in the form of grain, and our teeth are not structured to chew them. To be more precise, cereals in nature are often found because they are cultivated by humans and not because there is spontaneous growth. Anything that is artificially derived from nature's offer is not covered by the paleo diet.

The paleo diet is based on the intake of fibrous carbohydrates (fruits and vegetables in large quantities), fats (seeds and berries) and in small proportion proteins (fish or small animals).

The benefits that this diet possesses are undeniable: it is useful for those who are overweight, for those suffering from diabetes, high blood sugar, cardiovascular and degenerative diseases. It is assumed that one of the healthiest foods such as cereals is eliminated: they are in fact the main culprits of an increase in blood glucose within the blood. We often underestimate the fact that carbohydrates, useful for the body, are found in vegetables in greater quantities than cereals.

Reverse Disease, Stay Fit and Improve your Lifestyle

The paleo diet is a diet - even if for its supporters it is a real lifestyle - according to which only the foods that our ancestors ate in the Paleolithic era were consumed. This means that it is based not only on fruit and vegetables but also on fish, meat, roots and dried fruit, products that are believed to provide the necessary amount of antioxidants, minerals and vitamins, and protein. In principle, nutrients should be distributed in such a way as to consume between 20 and 35% of proteins, between 30 and 45% of lipids and between 20 and 40% of carbohydrates. However, there are some indications to respect: vegetables and fruit, for example, must be grown organically and naturally in season, just as animals must be raised on pasture.

As you can guess, the paleo diet excludes many of the foods we are used to consuming every day, including legumes, dairy products, cereals, sugar, sweets, and snacks of industrial production. The proponents of this theory believe that man has not had the time to evolve and to change his organism to be able to tolerate such foods, which have become part of human habits in a very recent era of evolutionary history. Since from the genetic point of view there are no differences between the man of today and that of 60 thousand years ago, here is that the paleo diet is more than enough to satisfy the needs of the organism.

The benefits that are guaranteed by this diet are obvious and easy to guess if you think that it excludes ingredients that, in fact, should still be taken in moderation: it is the case of dairy products and sugar, but also snacks, chips of all the savory snacks. Furthermore, it is recommended to consume organic fruits and vegetables, dried fruit and meat from animals raised in the wild: who could ever think that such foods are bad? Even fish should come from unpolluted water and be fished using traditional methods.

A direct consequence of the paleo diet, according to its fans, is the improvement of the digestive function: since our intestines host the four-fifths of our immune system, it is evident that if we consume foods every day that the body is not able to tolerate the digestive tract ends up becoming inflamed. Furthermore, with this dietary style there is the opportunity to intervene in the presence of sugar in the blood: knowing the quantity of carbohydrates, fats and proteins that it is necessary to take according to the needs of the organism, we eat once every 6 hours without being hit by the pangs of fame and allowed to be attracted by sweets or snacks. Moreover, and hydrogenated oils, even partially.

- **Weight Loss:** A high carbohydrate diet will make you gain a lot of weight - which is why so many people are overweight or obese. With the Paleo diet, you consume very little carbohydrate, but you focus on fat. The fatter your body consumes, the easier it will be to burn. This includes both the dietary fat you absorb and the fat already stored in your body.

- **Less Unhealthy Food:** If you've been interested in the food you have in your fridge and cupboard, you've probably been surprised by the number of unhealthy foods you've found there. White flour, white rice, sweets, pastries, baked goods, and other high-sugar products are just some of the foods you will give up on your Paleo diet. You will only eat foods that are good for your health.

- **Reduced Heart Problems:** Health problems are very often a result of our diet, and modern diets almost always lead to nutritional imbalances. With a paleo diet, you get back to basics, and you will see that the food you eat contains more nutrients that your body needs to stay healthy. You will have a healthier diet, and you will be healthier and have fewer problems!

- **Fewer Allergies:** Millions of people suffer from gluten sensitivity, lactose intolerance, and allergic reactions to grains, sugars, and other processed foods. By removing these foods from your diet, you remove the allergens that cause these reactions. You will feel healthier, more fit, especially because you will not have to fight against those allergens that have plagued you for years.

- **Fully Customizable Diet**: With the Paleo diet, there is no limit to the amount of food you can eat, only the foods you can eat. If you want to consume a healthy number of calories - that is, between 2000 and 2500 per day - you will have no strict guidelines to follow in terms of the amount and timing of your meals.

- **High in Nutrients:** When you're on a paleo diet, you eat foods high in fiber, omega-3 fatty acids, protein, healthy fat, and low-glycemic carbohydrates. You also avoid foods high in cholesterol, sodium, and all artificial and processed foods. In general, you provide your body with all the vitamins and minerals it needs to function properly and to be healthy.

- **No Risk of Cravings:** When you go on a paleo diet, you remove all snacks - such as chips, brownies, cakes, candy bars, etc. By eating healthy and balanced foods that satisfy you until the next meal you have no risk of suffering from cravings.
- **More Energy:** The healthier foods you eat; the more energy you will have. All the artificial, refined and processed foods you still eat today are sapping your energy. Removing them from your diet will allow you to have a lot more energy. You will also find that you will be more enduring because your body will have more calories available to feed your body.

- Reduced risk of developing certain degenerative diseases (including cancer, type 2 diabetes, and neurological decline): this decline is related to lower carbohydrate intake and increased intake of fruits and vegetables (which are rich in antioxidants, vitamins, minerals, and phytonutrients).
- Decreased inflammatory pain (related to the improvement of the acid/base ratio and Omega-3/6 ratio).
- **Reduced Risk of Heart Disease:** this is made possible in particular by the superior intake of good monounsaturated fats and Omega-3 (from walnuts, avocados, olive oil, fish and meat from animals fed on 'grass).
- Reduction of blood pressure.
- Regulation of cholesterol.
- Regulation of blood glucose.
- Better quality of sleep.
- Rise in skin quality (which becomes clearer), better teeth health.
- Improvement of symptoms related to gluten intolerance, less risk of food allergy.
- The disappearance of digestion problems and reflux of acidity.
- Prevention of osteoporosis.
- Possible relief of certain autoimmune diseases (significant decrease in pain caused by these diseases). Autoimmunity is a process in which our immune system makes antibodies to attack our tissues or constituents.

- **Satiety:** the massive intake of plants fills the stomach without energy concerns since they have a low caloric density.
- Lean proteins (meat without skin or visible fat) also satiate you between meals and help maintain strong muscles, healthy bones, and an optimal immune system.

Workouts Become More Effective.

However, non-paleo foods have an inflammatory effect that can lead to the manifestation of autoimmune diseases, especially related to the thyroid. Within the paleo diet, the Paleo Autoimmune Protocol has been defined which further restricts the range of foods allowed. People with hypothyroidism, Hashimoto, endometriosis, and sclerosis are advised to follow this protocol in an iron way for at least three months, and then gradually reintegrate some foods.

The Paleo Autoimmune Protocol is proposed as an anti-inflammatory therapy which, together with specific drugs, some support supplements and healthy life, helps to normalize the hormone values and reactivate the normal thyroid function. Keep in mind, however, that the Paleo diet, and especially the Paleo Autoimmune Protocol, must be followed under constant medical supervision.

Conclusively, the beneficial effects of the Paleo diet on health far outweigh the sacrifices at the table that it imposes. And you won't even have to give up the pleasures of the palate! In fact, you can adapt your meals to this new diet, to the great satisfaction of your taste buds.

CPSIA information can be obtained
at www.ICGtesting.com
Printed in the USA
LVHW050628100221
678897LV00003B/486

9 781801 561006